Gentle Exercise

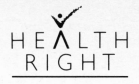

HEALTH RIGHT

Gentle Exercise
Susan Swire

J. M. Dent & Sons Ltd
London and Melbourne

First published 1986
© Susan Swire 1986

This book is set in 9½/10½pt Linotron 202 Times by
Book Economy Services, Sussex
Made in Great Britain by
Guernsey Press Co. Ltd, Guernsey, C.I.
for
J. M. Dent & Sons Ltd
Aldine House, 33 Welbeck Street, London W1M 8LX

British Library Cataloguing in Publication Data

Swire, Susan
  Gentle exercise.
  1. Exercise   2. Physical fitness
  I. Title
  613.7'1   RA781

  ISBN O-460-02449-3

CONTENTS

For my parents

INTRODUCTION

This book is for everyone, no matter what their age or level of fitness, who would like their body to be more supple and harmonious, to feel better and to look better.

Gentle Exercise makes it easy. First, it describes the norms of strength, alignment and flexibility for each part of the body in turn. These norms are not necessarily averages taking the population as a whole. They are the *optimum* for which everybody's joints are designed in order to render the body mobile yet stable. The simple exercises in these pages – almost all of them anaerobic – will then show you how to work swiftly, and safely, towards these ideals. They place equal emphasis on movements which *strengthen* (firm, tone up) the muscles and those which *stretch* (relax) them, giving suppleness, so that the whole body is brought into balance. Finally, *Gentle Exercise* is full of hints about vital principles of posture, breathing and relaxation which not only form the basis for the exercises themselves but, carried into everyday life, will have a transforming effect on emotional and psychological well-being as well as on general health and appearance.

The question, then, is simply one of knowing what we should be able to expect of ourselves and how best to help. Muscles adapt to the use that is made of them. They respond to increased work with better performance. If they are under-used, they deteriorate. The lengths of the muscles eventually adapt to habitual under-use or misuse. They can become chronically shortened or stretched, affecting the posture and making it impossible to move freely. Even feelings build themselves into our bodies. If we continually raise our shoulders with anxiety they hunch and thicken, and cannot fall into their natural elegant line. The arms will be clumsy and awkward. Worse, our anxiety is consolidated, and becomes repressed into our very structure.

It is not, of course, only muscles which adapt. Other soft tissue structures adapt in turn, though much more slowly, crystallizing the changes and casting the body in a less harmonious mould. Even bone in time responds to the habitual pull of the muscles upon it.

Yet this very malleability can be made to work *for* us, instead of being allowed to work against us. Not only is it possible to maintain the mobility that we have, it is also possible to regain what we have lost. The remarkable recoveries sometimes made by people after accidents are usually achieved by exercise – not the random flailings and contortions which comprise many a well intentioned workout, but precise movements tailored to specific difficulties. How much easier it must be, then, for those unscathed by illness or injury to overcome the minor muscular imbalances to which most people fall prey.

The primary cause – and cure – usually lies in the muscles, and since fortunately we have conscious control over our muscles, we have control too over our mobility and ultimately to some extent our shape. Moreover, while deterioration even in the cells is often reversible, this reversibility is particularly marked and rapid in the muscles. We cannot help the bones and ligaments directly. With exercise we *can* help the muscles. Other structures tend to adapt accordingly.

The exercises here form a balanced selection of those I taught in two of Britain's leading health farms, and ultimately derive from the methods often used in the rehabilitation of accident and arthritis victims. My background in exercise is orthodox, that of a chartered physiotherapist. My interests have extended to complementary medicine and alternative techniques, and particularly to systems such as t'ai chi ch'uan, yoga and the Alexander Technique. I have studied under teachers in Britain, India and California. From my work with patients in hospitals I learnt the necessity of gaining results quickly and safely, always using sound anatomical principles. From yoga and t'ai chi came the appreciation of flow and balance and of slow slow movement. From Alexander we learn the sense of alignment in everything we do. These old/new, East/West sources gave birth to the exercises in this book which together form a holistic system blending softness with strength. They are for you to explore. And to enjoy.

Acknowledgments

I should like particularly to thank Jennie Elston and John Tindall who acted as models for the exercise photographs. They demonstrate so beautifully what everyone can aim to achieve.

Before You Begin

THE FUNDAMENTALS

Posture

'Good posture' can bring to mind something stiff, immobile, unnatural — a static position rather than a dynamic pattern. But whenever we consider our posture we ought to think in terms of flow and balance, constantly shifting and adjusting but 'all of a piece' — stillness in action.

The ideal posture is one in which minimum effort and energy are expended for maximum efficiency and endurance. Everyone's body is individual, and exact alignment will vary slightly from person to person. But there are functional and aesthetic ideals which can act as guidelines. The further we deviate from the accepted norms the more work the muscles must do just to maintain our balance. In fact, in a standing position most of the muscles should do very little, as the ligaments provide the primary support.

The line of gravity is an imaginary plumb-line which passes through the centre of gravity or balancing point. (In the human standing position the centre of gravity is a couple of inches below the navel, but deep inside the body.) The more centrally the gravity line falls within the base (the feet and the area between them), the more stable and balanced the body. The more it nears the edge of the base, the more unstable it is and the harder the muscles must work just to maintain the balance. Ideally, when standing, the line of gravity is such that the three big weight masses of the body — pelvis, ribcage and head — will line up vertically over one another. The 'plumb-line' will fall from the crown of the head to just in front of the ankle bones, with the bodyweight equally balanced between the heels and the balls of the feet. The nose will be in line with the navel, the lobes of the ears with the points of the shoulders.

The effects of improved posture are transforming. You will feel more poised and tranquil. You can look up to 10 pounds slimmer, looser limbed, more svelte. Your abdomen will be firmer, your waistline neater. Breathing deepens, food is better assimilated.

Eyesight often improves. Throughout these pages you will find many tips to help you. First let us consider the basic concepts of grounding, centring, growth and expansion.

Grounding

Are your feet on the ground or is your head in the clouds? Do you stand on your own two feet or do you lean on others? Can you hold your ground or are you easily thrown? Our language speaks in metaphors but the body images it uses are very real. The body and the psyche are inextricably linked.

From a mechanical point of view the stability of any object depends on three factors: the base of support, the line of gravity in relation to the base, and the centre of gravity. The larger the base, the closer the line of gravity to the middle of the base, and the lower the centre of gravity, the better the balance.

The base of support is crucial to equilibrium. Standing upright, our base is small in relation to our height. This has given us certain benefits of mobility at the expense of stability. It is therefore of the greatest importance that optimum advantage is made of the base we have. We need to be 'grounded'. Today, many of us live in our head. Our whole culture encourages us to do so. Our education almost guarantees it. This is both a physical and a psychological state. Almost everyone, when asked where in the body they feel their *self* to be, points to the head or upper chest. The problem is one of imbalance. We hold ourselves up out of our base, overemphasizing the upper part of our body.

Our legs support us. The earth sustains us. We need to give them proper attention, for no structure is stronger than its foundation. Feel the earth beneath your feet. Let your body-weight sink down into it. Allow your tensions to drain through your legs and feet to be absorbed by it. When you walk, give the whole of your weight to the supporting foot. When you sit, feel the contact of your sitting bones with the ground or chair. Your base will then be firm and stable.

The change is small, merely a shift of attention, but the psychophysical benefits are immense. The sections on the feet, knees and hips are devoted to these foundations, and it is because this sense of grounding is basic to balance that the exercises in the book proceed from the feet up.

Centring

The centre of gravity is the imaginary point in a body around which all the surrounding masses are equal — the point of balance. It is easy to visualize it in a round ball as being the very centre, the point which is equidistant from every part of the surface. In the human being the centre of gravity in the standing position is, as we have noted, just below the navel and deep inside. The exact location varies somewhat according to the shape and position of the body. It is an inch or so higher in men (with their more powerful shoulders) than in women (with their broader hips). In certain movements it can even lie outside the body. If with just one fingertip you press someone on their sacrum (the flat bone at the bottom of the back) on a level with their centre of gravity they will step forward. If you press from the side at the appropriate level they will move sideways. Very light pressure from behind can be used to help a weak person to walk.

Since in the human body the centre, at 50-55 per cent of total body height above the ground, is quite high, it is again important to optimize our structure as it is. Most of us, however, act as though the pivot point is still higher. We are not 'centred'. We hold ourselves up from our chest. Many people feel the greatest area of tension in the body to be just behind the breastbone. It is as if we would crumple if we did not hang on from above. By 'holding up' with the emphasis on the upper part of the body we are effectively raising our centre of gravity, making our body less stable. Again, only a shift of attention is needed. While remaining grounded, at one with the earth, be aware of your own primal centre deep inside you. Drop down into it. Be centred there.

The centre is the foundation of stable posture. If you turn to the right or the left, turn from your centre not from your shoulders. The movement will then be effortless. If you step forward, proceed from your centre. If you climb stairs, let your centre propel you up. Speak from your centre too. Your voice will be warm and mellow and without the harsh edge of a voice that comes from the chest or throat.

The Chinese and Japanese have long held the concept of 'the centre' to be the spiritual as well as the mechanical centre of our being. In hara kiri, the Japanese ritual suicide by disembowelling, the belly was chosen because to the Japanese it is the seat of life.

There is a similar notion in Judaism called 'Jerusalem'. In the West we speak of the 'still small centre'. As the centre of gravity is the basis of balanced posture and movement, so it is the basis of psychological balance. The centred person acquires an inner resilience which makes it possible to face life calmly and to be prepared for anything. It has even been claimed that a dropping down into our true centre actually heightens the senses, expanding the perceptions and increasing our enjoyment of the world around us. The centre of a ball stays in the same relationship to the periphery however the ball rolls. The hub of a wheel maintains its centre as the spokes and rim revolve. The centre of the cyclone is still. The heart of the whirlpool is undisturbed. Find your own still small centre. Let your life emanate from there.

The abdominal and back exercises given here will not make you centred. Only a dropping of your awareness into your centre will do that. They will, however, help restore or maintain its tone and elasticity.

Growth and Expansion

Grounding and centring are also fundamental to the poise of the head and the freedom of the arms. Sink your weight into your feet, or into your sitting bones when you are seated. Find your centre. Then, and only then, consider your upper body. Visualize your plumb-line, your line of gravity, as a puppet's thread suspending you from the crown (back) of the head. Let it lengthen and straighten the back of your neck. Your neck will then be free. Imagine a weight on the end of your spine pulling your tailbone down, away from the point of suspension above, so your backbone can lengthen. Grounding and centring combined with the 'uplift' can change your whole awareness to a very satisfying one of solidity and support below and lightness and freedom above. If you are not grounded and centred any upward orientation leaves you, like the puppet, 'scattered'.

The sections on the neck and shoulders contain many hints for gaining poise and openness in the upper body. But these are only valid in conjunction with a solid 'ground' and a firm 'centre'. If you are grounded and centred you are free to explore and reach out in any direction and yet maintain equilibrium — to expand, grow and be creative.

Breathing

Before food, even before water, sustenance comes from the air we breathe. Oxygen is the primary nourishment of the cells. It is extracted from the air we inhale and carried by the bloodstream to every cell in the body. Similarly, breathing is the main mechanism for ridding the body of its toxins. The cells return waste carbon dioxide to the blood, and it is transported back to the lungs and exhaled with the other unwanted gases.

Health and emotional state are intimately linked with breathing. It is vital to breathe properly and in this the body knows best what is needed. Each person's respiration is tied to the demands of their own system at any given moment. The way we breathe has an immediate effect on our biochemistry and mood. Personally, I am against breathing 'exercises' unless one understands exactly what one is doing. No arbitrarily imposed breathing technique will perfectly match the cells' delicately balanced moment-to-moment requirements. All interference with the natural rhythm has its effect. If one hyperventilates one can become lightheaded or faint. Breathing in certain ways is sometimes deliberately used to induce abreactions, even the re-experiencing of birth (as in rebirthing techniques). It can help open doors to psychic worlds. Before starting to manipulate your breathing it is wise to be clear just what you are aiming for, physically and psychologically.

The way many people habitually breathe is not conducive to optimum health and tranquillity, for they often interfere subconsciously with their natural rhythm. By far the most common breathing problem is to emphasize the inbreath, never fully letting go of the stale air. When we are anxious we often hold our breath tightly, hardly releasing the air at all. These tendencies are exaggerated in chest conditions such as bronchitis and asthma and can lead to a stiff neck and shoulders, eyestrain and raised blood pressure. Breath retention is a major cause of fatigue as toxic wastes are stockpiled in the body. With raised levels of carbon dioxide in the blood the brain is stimulated so that the person tends to be irritable and over-reactive.

Check your own breathing. Are you holding your breath just a fraction? If so drop your shoulders and with a sigh of relief let the air go. Observe yourself whenever you are upset. If you find yourself clinging to the air you will be surprised how much easier it is to cope once you let it free.

Perhaps breath-holding is a maladaptive development of a useful protective response in the animal kingdom. A rabbit may 'play dead' if it is frightened. It then stops breathing and lies still as a stone. The fox goes on its way in search of more animated quarry. The rabbit, safe again, breathes and scampers on. When we meet anxiety we re-enact this primal pattern. We hold our breath and anaesthetize ourselves. For human beings the response is counterproductive for, thus paralysed, we cannot react appropriately. Many of us in fact exhibit some degree of breath-holding all the time. It is a habit we learn early. Babies sometimes hold their breath quite alarmingly in response to unwanted stimuli. Many breathing exercises only exaggerate the problem, emphasizing the intake of air. We 'open the window and breathe *in* the fresh air' with a great heave of the chest. Other exercises which try to overcome this bias ('breathe in for seven paces and out for ten') are quite arbitrary, taking no account of the body's own intrinsic rhythms.

What we often think of as deep breathing, the forced exaggerated expansion of the upper chest, is in fact shallow breathing making use only of the upper areas of the lungs. Instead of dictating to your body, simply *observe* your breathing. Tune in to your own rhythm. Allow it to happen. Be aware of the inflow and the outflow. Drop your shoulders. Let the air go completely. Do not *make* it go. Just allow all your tension to flow away with your breath. And wait. Wait for the air to come in. It will come of its own accord.

As we watch and wait, the breathing changes subtly. The ribs and abdomen expand as the air comes in and fall back into place as the air flows away. They expand much more than before. The breathing becomes naturally deeper and slower. We feel calmer and quieter. Detached awareness of one's breathing can be used as a meditation technique. Nothing more is needed. Just watch the rise and fall of the breath. Let yourself be 'breathed'.

This allowing of the breath rather than a controlling of it is carried over into the exercises. 'Breathe easily' is written into the exercise instructions. Never forget to allow the air to come and go during the exercises. Especially let it go. If you *do* breathe freely and naturally instead of holding your breath, your muscles should not ache after these gentle exercises.

Relaxation

Being able to relax is an invaluable asset. It is impossible to feel anxiety if your body is totally relaxed. There are numerous techniques of relaxation, but the important factor is to be able to carry the relaxation over into the stressful situations of everyday life. This section will concentrate on a few hints for relaxation that do not require you to be still or alone or cocooned in a peaceful environment. They will help switch off the fright/fight/flight mechanism and switch on rest/relaxation/recuperation.

First of all, remember everything which has been said in this chapter so far. Observe your breathing. Ground yourself. Visualize your bodyweight draining down, seeping into all the surfaces that support you, and flowing down too into those parts of your body that are unsupported. Together, grounding, centring and easy balance of the head will dissipate much of the excess tension of everyday activity. Your body relaxes because it is in equilibrium and has no unnecessary work to do.

Then release the stress positions. Uncross your legs. Release your abdomen. Drop your shoulders. Unfold your arms — do not let your upper arms squeeze in to hug your body. Unclench your hands — do not allow them to clutch at each other; let the fingertips do all the work so that the arms are loose and free. Imagining your head suspended from the crown, let the back of your neck be long and straight; your chin will then be level and not poking up. Let your eyes and mouth be soft; do not clench your teeth or purse your lips; release your tongue if you are holding it rigidly against the roof of your mouth; imagine your eyes are very wide apart and let them be mobile, not fixed or staring. Let your bodyweight fall just in front of your ankle bones.

Do the stretching exercises in this book. Tense muscles are short muscles. When you stretch them very slowly you relax them. You can see from the exercise subheadings which the stretching exercises are. If they are difficult it is likely that you have localized tension in the particular muscles concerned, and such tension is often part of a pattern of general tension. The stretching of tense shortened muscles can be quite painful. It feels anything but relaxing. However, a strong feeling of pull *in the muscles* indicates the stretching (relaxing) of tense areas. You can minimize pain and maximize the relaxation by stretching on the outbreaths.

Tension is a muscular state, but since there are no nerve endings to register tension in the muscles, the brain cannot recognize or affect what is going on in them. It is a waste of time therefore to lie on your back hypnotically intoning: '*Relax* your calves. *Relax* your thighs. *Relax* your buttocks', etc. To relax muscles they must be lengthened by releasing positions of stress or by actually stretching with exercise.

Some kinds of psychological approach may, however, be beneficial. One visualization technique, warm abdomen and cool forehead, is taught by doctors and other health professions in the Autogenic Training method of stress reduction. Whoever heard of a relaxed hothead? If you keep a cool head you remain calm and relaxed. Compare this with the ancient Tibetan practice of visualizing the chest area as cool, a technique which, it is claimed, lowers body temperature and prolongs life.

Another idea is pure 'fringe', but it is worth trying. To relax and protect yourself if you are frightened or in danger, imagine you are wearing a silver cloak, a cloak with a hood, enveloping you from head to foot, a cloak as soft and silver as the stars. This secret was given to me by a mystically inclined Russian princess.

Finally, be kind to yourself. Skilled massage can be a great help in relaxing taut muscles and minds. If muscles are chronically tight, as for example they frequently are in the neck and shoulders, deep massage can be quite painful, but it is good pain, which releases as soon as the tension starts to dissipate. It is worth indulging yourself from time to time.

ABOUT GENTLE EXERCISE

The Exercises

Exercise can be a waste of time without some clear objective. The important thing is to understand your own particular physique and to be aware of any muscular imbalance you may have. The illustrations at the beginning of each section demonstrate the optimum alignment for every part of the body and state just how much movement there should be in each joint. They show which exercise helps achieve which ideal by normalizing the length and tone of the muscles which act on the specific joint.

Exercises are at best artificial. They cannot replace normal healthy activity — walking, swimming, dancing and the like — but carefully chosen they can help your performance in any of these things. Basically, they have three functions — they improve strength, suppleness, and stamina. No exercise maximally achieves all three ends at once, and the emphasis in this book is on strength and suppleness. The exercises form an integrated system which helps bring the whole body into equilibrium, tightening slack areas and relaxing tense, tight ones. As a result the body is gradually reshaped along more pleasing lines, allowing better coordination and greater freedom and economy of movement.

The instructions for each exercise tell you not only what to do, but how to do it to best effect and why it may be useful. It is a good idea to concentrate first on the areas where there is restriction and bring them into balance with the rest of the body. Eventually, all the exercises should be equally easy.

Strengthening and stretching exercises are given for each muscle group in turn except where they would be inappropriate. (Nobody wants to overstretch their throat and create a double chin, or slacken their bottom or their abdomen.) Strengthening and stretching are equally important. The stretches increase suppleness, but suppleness should not be emphasized at the expense of strength because the joints can become unstable. Nor is there any virtue in massive strength if it involves loss of flexibility. The aim should be to keep the two in balance. It is not a good idea to follow a system which promotes only stretching or only strengthening.

Strength and Suppleness

The degree of *strength* aimed at in these exercises is that which you need for good posture and for the demands of everyday activity, plus a little reserve. It is achieved by lifting the bodyweight against gravity. To increase one's strength more than this, weights (or some other form of resistance such as manual resistance) must be used, preferably stepping up the weight and number of repeats scientifically. Many of the strengthening exercises in this book can be adapted for gentle weight-lifting. In the leg lifts, for example, you can attach a weight to your ankle. The muscles have to work harder to lift the leg and are strengthened accordingly. Gradually you can increase the weight and/or the number of repetitions.

The degree of *suppleness* aimed for is the accepted normal range of movement of each individual joint as shown at the beginning of each section. It is achieved by the muscle-stretching exercises, performed slowly and with awareness. The slow holding at the limit of movement is the secret of restoring suppleness, the secret that has always been exploited by yoga. Apart from the feeling of well-being the muscle stretches give once you can do them easily, they have the very real value of making you less vulnerable to injury. A flexible body is more resilient. A flexible *strong* body is even less susceptible to injury. The stretches also release tension from the muscles and so set free a great deal of energy which may previously have been bound up. Muscular and energy release can then bring about emotional release.

Isometric or Isotonic?

Muscles can work 'isotonically' or 'isometrically'. The prefix 'iso' means 'the same'. 'Tonic' relates to muscle tone and 'metric' to muscle length. When working isotonically the muscle *tone* remains the same but the length alters. When working isometrically, the *length* stays the same but the tone is increased. An easy way to visualize this is to think of the muscles which span the top of the shoulder to the upper arm. They must contract or shorten to lift the arm up. The two ends or attachments of the muscles draw closer together. To lower the arm in a controlled way the muscles must still work, otherwise the arm would just drop to the side. Here the muscle attachments are drawn apart by gravity. The muscles lengthen. In both cases the length changes but the muscle tone stays the same. The muscle work is isotonic. To hold the arm in mid-air the muscles stay the same length. Their tone increases. They now work isometrically.

Isometric exercise therefore is static. The muscles contract but there is no movement. Pushing loads and carrying are isometric. Isotonic exercise, on the other hand, indicates movement. Swimming and dancing are isotonic.

Fashions come and go in exercise as in everything, and a recent vogue was 'isometrics' or 'how to get strong without moving a muscle'. Isometric exercise builds strength in the muscles being worked (provided the intensity of the muscle contraction is over 80 per cent of the muscle's maximum strength). Squeezing a tennis ball hard for a couple of seconds many times a day, for instance, will quite dramatically increase the strength of the arm muscles responsible for the flexing and gripping action of the fingers. The advantage of isometrics is that they require hardly any time or space. Anyone can do them, any time, any where. Therapeutically, isometric exercise has been found useful for strengthening and building bulk in wasted muscles where movement is difficult or impossible — after operations or recent injuries perhaps, or where there is too much pain.

However, isometric exercise should be treated with caution. It can cause a massive increase in blood pressure. (Clenching your fist can help avert a faint if you feel one coming on.) Unlike isotonic (movement) exercise, it has no benign pumping action on the circulation. An isometrically overworked muscle can be depleted of its necessary nutriments and saturated with its own waste products so that it eventually stops working. At best it will ache quite badly the following day. Although, like isotonic exercise, isometrics can strengthen muscles, they cannot relax localized tension or increase general body endurance. For these reasons most of the exercises in this book are isotonic.

Isometric exercise — whether as 'exercises' or in daily life — should always be interspersed with plenty of free movement.

Because of the effect on the blood pressure, muscle contractions should not be held for too long. I usually suggest several contractions of six seconds with complete relaxation between holds. And, for the same reason, it is very important not to hold your breath. Let it come and go naturally. Allow the outbreath.

Aerobic or Anaerobic?

If isometrics was something of a fad a while ago, aerobics have recently become an obsession — as well as big business. Of course nothing is new and we have been doing aerobics ever since we were thrown out of Eden to toil for a living. Now the living is a little too soft, and undoubtedly some supplementary aerobic exercise is essential for good health.

'Aerobic' means with oxygen. 'Anaerobic' means without oxygen. Aerobic exercise is activity which is taxing enough to make you breathe more deeply. It improves the efficiency of the heart, lungs and circulation, and increases the total blood volume. All aerobic work involves the legs, which help pump the blood back to the heart to provide the body with more oxygen with which to produce energy. Jogging is aerobic as, in its gentle way, is t'ai chi. Anaerobic exercise, such as weightlifting or yoga, works directly on the muscles.

Of the three major benefits from exercise — increased stamina, strength and suppleness — it is stamina primarily which is improved by aerobic exercise. Appropriate anaerobic exercise promotes strength and suppleness. Aerobic exercise trains the system to sustain prolonged strenuous activity. Anaerobic exercise can help the muscles to withstand it. This book concentrates mainly on anaerobic exercises, done slowly and thoughtfully. (A selection of the same exercises performed vigorously could of course be combined into an aerobic workout, though much of their specific benefit would be lost.)

Since no single activity maximally improves strength, supple-ness *and* stamina one should, ideally, have some aerobic as well as some proper anaerobic exercise daily. Many natural activities will provide an adequate amount of aerobic exercise. Running, cycling, swimming, dancing, even walking will make you feel better, healthier, more alive. Skipping is excellent. Perhaps the most valuable of the 'artificial' aerobic exercises is bouncing on a mini-trampoline (see no.10). Once you have the bouncer (trampoline) it costs you nothing. It is quick, easy and fun, especially if you bounce to music.

Aerobics classes themselves can be marvellous, but they are not without their hazards. As with all exercise classes, make sure your teacher is properly trained (for example, is a qualified P.E. teacher or physiotherapist), and that he or she understands enough about the body — your body. Every physiotherapist will have had to deal with damage resulting from overenthusiastic or unwise exercises, both aerobic and anaerobic. I recently treated an aerobics teacher who had jumped and jolted and jarred so much that her feet had seized up altogether.

Fifteen minutes of continuous aerobic exercise done three times a week is said to maintain fitness. Six times a week will substantially increase it. (These figures are quoted from the literature of one of the mini-trampoline makers. Other sources stipulate rather lower requirements.) What is important is that you start slowly — maybe two or three minutes or less — and build up gradually.

There are elaborate methods of pulse-taking to calculate just how much aerobic exercise is right for you at any given time, but all that is really necessary is that you use your common sense. Do some gentle rhythmic warm-ups first. Build up slowly. The essence of aerobic exercise is that you breathe more deeply. But stop if you are puffed. If you are too out of breath to hold a conversation you have done far too much. Stop if, or before, you are dizzy. Stop long before you have a pain in your chest. Don't exercise at all if you are too tired or have any infection. 'Feeling the burn' means the muscle has used its oxygen and is dying. Do *not* go for the burn. Enjoy your aerobics. Have fun, but listen to your body. Do not let anybody — anybody at all — force you.

Improvement or Maintenance?

To *restore* optimum mobility where it is lacking requires work on the appropriate exercises. Take them to your present limit — and that little bit more. It is that little bit more which facilitates fluid, graceful movement and a more elastic body. Explore your limits and push them back just a little each day. Always avoid straining, however, by breathing easily and allowing the outbreath. As the aim is to bring the body into balance, if you find any movement more difficult or restricted on one side than the other, work harder on the weaker or stiffer side.

To *maintain* movement which is already free, the ideal is to take each joint through its full range of movement once a day. But there is no point in becoming fanatical. That way you only become tense and undo much of the benefit. Practise when you can.

Selected exercises can thus be used to free restricted movement in specific parts of the body. Together they can be used as a lifetime maintenance programme.

Progression

These exercises are based on pure anatomical movements, the basic building blocks of all movement (which in real life are combined and modified into *patterns* of movement). They reduce muscle work to its simplest, most specific actions. Because of this, and because they are done slowly without any sudden jolting, they are both self-limiting (safe) and self-progressing.

With practice you do more, get further into each movement. You do as much as you can today. You do more tomorrow. The exercises act so specifically that results are gained quickly. Eventually all the movements become easy. You can then use them as a body maintenance programme or as limbering for any sport or physical activity.

Provided you breathe easily and take note of the cautions, you cannot hurt yourself. Age is no barrier and it is a fact that older people often progress more quickly than younger, apparently fitter, ones. These movements are based on those taught in hospital physiotherapy departments where the physical ability of people of all ages suffering a variety of injuries and illnesses is very mixed. You cannot go beyond your present limit (and of course that little bit more), and until you have mastered a movement it is hard work whatever your general condition.

It is important to stress, however, that if you have any doubt at all about your physical state, or if you are pregnant, you should seek professional medical advice before embarking on these, or any other, exercises.

Visualization

It will help if you visualize yourself performing with ease the movement you are aiming for. We create our bodies (and many other aspects of our lives) not only by direct intervention but also through the imagination. There is evidence that visualization can radically affect performance. In one study, by the psychologist Alan Richardson, Richardson chose three groups of people at random and measured their performance at basketball free-throw shooting. For twenty days, the first group spent twenty minutes a day practising free throws; the second group did not practise at all; the third group spent twenty minutes a day visualizing themselves scoring free throws. At the end of the twenty days the first group had improved by 24 per cent, the second group had not improved at all, and the third group, the visualizers, had improved by 23 per cent. It is a pity that there does not appear to have been a fourth group, who practised *and* visualized. It would seem, however, that creative visualization is not a substitute for action, but that it can reinforce it immensely. (Experiments with dart throwing and other activities have shown similar results.)

The secret of successful visualization is to relax, to let go, to breathe freely and spontaneously. In the normal active waking state the brain registers beta waves. When we relax, the brain waves change and slow down to an alpha rhythm, which has been found to be far more effective in creating real changes in the so-called objective world.

Strain and Pain

When doing the exercises you should feel no strain or pain in your back or joints. A strong sustained sensation of pull in the *muscles* (e.g. the calves) is perfectly acceptable provided you relax into the stretch, little by little. Usually a greater muscle stretch is possible on the outbreaths, so use these to gain extra movement. (Never, however, allow any interference with your normal breathing pattern. Use the outbreaths or the inbreaths *as they happen* to gain the extra stretching or strengthening effect.) These exercises are almost all performed very slowly. Always avoid sudden sharp stretches as they can have the reverse effect by stimulating the stretch reflex, the mechanism which makes muscles contract still further to protect the body against overstretch.

Between each exercise, or each repetition of an exercise, release all the residual tension from the previous movement. Drop your shoulders. Breathe easily and relax. Start afresh each time.

There should never be *any* residual pain immediately the exercise position is released (although there may well be muscle stiffness the following day, especially if you held your breath during the exercise). Distinguish between the hurt that helps (stretch of shortened muscles) and the hurt that can harm (in your back and joints).

None of the movements in the following pages is contortionist. They aim merely to help you to maintain or attain the alignment and freedom of movement which is everybody's natural right. When you can perform every exercise easily you will indeed be in balance.

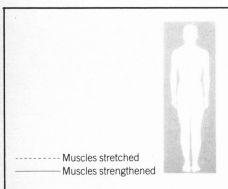

------- Muscles stretched
——— Muscles strengthened

Numbers in bold type indicate exercises which will help correct the relevant postural fault or achieve the appropriate range of movement. One or more muscles may be at fault in certain instances. This is why in some cases so many exercises have been suggested.

The Exercises

WARM-UPS

Warm-ups are easy, rhythmic movements which help limber you up prior to more strenuous exercise by stimulating the circulation and easing the muscles into activity. The essence of warm-ups is that they are relaxed and gentle. Unlike exercises proper you are not aiming to take yourself to your limits or push back barriers. Any rhythmic pendular or circular movements will do. Simple swinging of your legs, for example, will help prepare your leg and hip muscles. Here are a few 'all-over' exercises which will leave you refreshed and exhilarated.

1 Stretch, Yawn, Blink

Stretch your arms out as far as you can. Yawn. Blink a few times. Breathe easily. (Repeat.)

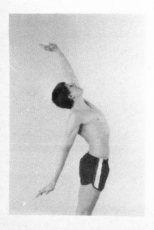

Think of a cat stretching slowly, sensuously. When it wakes up, it stretches its limbs. It stretches its back. It yawns. It takes its time. Be like a cat. Stretch your arms — out, up, behind you, as far as they will go. Twist them first in one direction, then another. Feel your back becoming part of the stretch. Sense your neck elongating. Let your legs take part. Enjoy the stretch. At the same time, yawn. Usually, thinking about a yawn is enough to bring one on. The stretch itself often produces a yawn. To simulate a yawn, stretch your arms, drop your jaw and take a deep breath in. Hold and suddenly let go. You will probably find yourself overtaken by a deep refreshing yawn. After the yawn, blink a few times — the softest, lightest blinks possible. Give yourself a moment or two to savour the feeling of release that this exercise gives you.

The Benefit
This is the best, most natural wake-up exercise possible. Do it first thing in the morning; before your exercises; any time you feel the need to revive yourself. The *stretching* increases the circulation to every part of the body. It activates and limbers the muscles. *Yawning* is a reflex action which happens whenever we are tired or bored, or when there is too much carbon dioxide in the blood. It happens, for some reason which is not properly understood, when we see someone else yawn. Yawning helps bring the chemistry of the blood back into balance and imparts a sense of freshness. It also stimulates the tear ducts and moistens the eyes with the fluid they need to remain healthy. Rather than stifling yawns we should encourage them and yawn frequently. *Blinking* also helps lubricate and brighten the eyes. It rests them momentarily from their constant job of seeing. Provided the blinks are soft and light, not harsh or tense, the eyesight may become temporarily clearer.

If you do not do another single thing in this book, remember to stretch, yawn and lightly blink.

2 Limbering Rock

Sit, knees bent, chin on chest, hands clasped around legs — curled in a little ball. Roll backward and forward in one smooth movement. Breathe easily. (Repeat.)

Aim for a smooth backward and forward rock with no pause on your head and shoulders. You should, however, be able to stop dead when you return to the sitting position. The secret lies in staying in a little ball — chin tucked in, knees close to you, and in remaining 'centred'. Feel every single part of your spine as it comes into contact with the ground, being aware especially of the vertebrae in the small of your back.

The Benefit
You will feel a pleasant exhilaration as your back is gently massaged and your circulation stimulated. The rocking requires and promotes coordination, strength and suppleness, and generates a feeling of well-being.

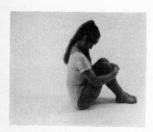

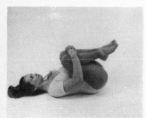

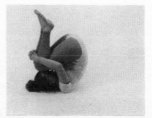

3 Limbering Roll

Lie on the floor, knees bent, chin on chest, hands clasped around legs — curled in a little ball. Breathe easily. Roll from side to side.

Stay curled up in a ball and roll slowly and gently from side to side without a pause. Control the movement so there is no jerking up or falling sideways — just a nice, smooth roll. Let your low back be in contact with the ground for the whole of the roll.

The Benefit
Providing you roll on your *low* back you will give yourself a wonderful massage — firm and soothing — nearly as nice as having someone else massage you (though it does not work if the small of your back loses contact with the ground). Rolling on your back is a delicious sensation. Remember how ecstatically a puppy rolls from side to side. Keeping your back down also helps to tone the abdominal muscles.

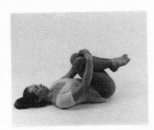

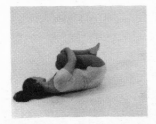

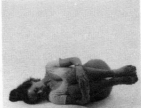

4 The Cat

Kneel on all fours, back straight, hands directly under your shoulders, knees a little way apart and directly under your hips. Drop your head to look between your knees and round your back as far as you can go. Return to the flat-back position and lift your head and your bottom. Move slowly and smoothly several times between one position and the other. Breathe easily.

Keep your arms and legs firm and at right-angles to the ground so that you do not sway back and forth. Your fingers should be pointing forwards and your elbows straight. As you lift your head and your bottom, make sure your midriff does not sag down too abruptly. This is a slow flowing motion, sinuous, continuous. There is no break, simply one wave-like action in which the limit of the one direction becomes the beginning of the next, without pause. Feel every joint of your spine as it alternately flexes and extends. Be aware of that instant in time when your back and neck are quite straight. It is a movement to enjoy. Think of a cat which stretches its back when it is content or arches it when it is angry. You can feel as graceful as the cat.

The Benefit
The alternate flexing and stretching will make your back beautifully supple, and the arching up will strengthen your abdominal muscles. The warmth you may feel along your spine is

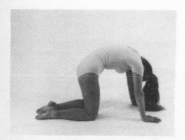
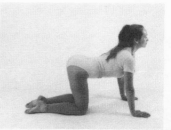

indicative of the increased circulation. Your whole system benefits from this exercise and, of them all, it is perhaps the nicest one to do.

Caution
If you have just had a baby, or if your abdominal muscles are extremely weak and are sagging badly, only come to the flat-back position. Do not lift your head and bottom or hollow your back until your abdominal muscles are stronger.

FOOTNOTES

(Foot, ankle, lower leg)

Straight, strong, supple feet are essential for smooth movement in the body as a whole. When standing and walking your feet should, first of all, be straight, parallel with one another. The real strain comes when they habitually point out, leading possibly to osteoarthritis of the feet, knees or hips. (Ballet dancers *look* beautiful, toes turned out, but are prone eventually to painful joint disorders.) Equally imbalanced, if less common, is a pigeon-toed stance with the toes turning in. Sometimes there is an inequality, one foot turning more than the other. Check what is happening and if need be straighten one or both feet. You may feel quite odd when you straighten them, but the muscles will quickly adapt. Practice constantly until the new position feels natural for you.

The heel and ball of each foot and the inside and outside should bear weight evenly. There are ideally three points of equal weightbearing — two on the ball of the foot, just behind the big and little toes, and a third in the centre of the heel.

To distribute weight evenly from *front to back*, rock gently backwards and forwards keeping your feet parallel and heels and toes on the ground. As you sway, become aware of the many possible variations. Slowly come to rest in your habitual posture. Is your bodyweight over your heels? A puff of wind could blow you over. Not for nothing do we call some people push-overs. Is your weight taken on your toes? Then you are stuck, unable to react to situations in a flexible manner. In the optimum alert yet relaxed stance, with the line of gravity falling just in front of the ankle bones, you will feel the weight evenly between the heels and balls of the feet. (It has been observed that women, culturally conditioned to be submissive, very commonly take their weight over their heels, sometimes with a backward lean of the whole body, whereas the thrusting position, forward over the toes, is seen more often in men.)

To distribute your weight evenly from *side to side*, stand with

The Ideal

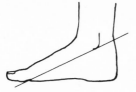

Normal long arch

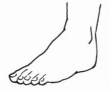

Normal metatarsal arch
Straight toes

feet parallel, the 'plumb-line' falling just in front of your ankle bones, and check your ankles. They should be upright, rolling neither in nor out. If the ankles collapse inwards they are weakened mechanically. Weight is thrust on to the big toes and inner borders of the feet in a way which is conducive to bunions and flat feet. Equally they should not bow out, with the bodyweight only on the outer borders of the feet. Like the supports of a bridge, your ankles have a weightbearing function. The outer and inner borders of the feet, including the big toes, should be in sensitive contact with the ground so that they play an equal part in taking your weight.

To help imbalanced distribution of weight it may also be necessary to correct the way you hold your knees. Your kneecaps, like your feet, should face directly ahead. If, when your feet are parallel, your knees turn in or out, swivel your thighs until your knees are quite straight. You may need a mirror for this. If you find it difficult, just bend your knees a little, adjust them in the bent position and stand up. Your kneecaps should now be looking straight ahead, your feet and legs firm and strong.

People who stand with their toes habitually turned out often find when they straighten their feet that their kneecaps become 'cross-eyed', rolling in to look at each other. The condition when your toes turn out and your kneecaps are straight, or feet straight but knees in, is known (inaccurately) as tibial torsion. Tibial torsion is associated with a great deal of mechanical strain — uneven weight distribution, possibly flat feet, maybe bunions. Flat feet, more often than not, are merely a functional problem resulting from postural deviation or imbalanced weightbearing, rather than a structural disorder. They can usually be corrected instantaneously.

Common Deviations

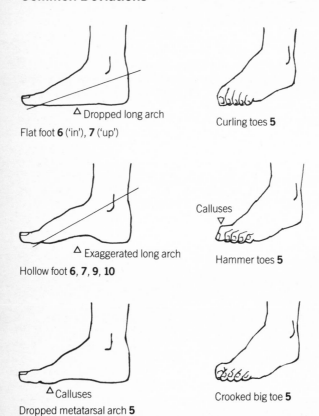

△ Dropped long arch

Flat foot **6** ('in'), **7** ('up')

Curling toes **5**

△ Exaggerated long arch

Hollow foot **6**, **7**, **9**, **10**

Calluses
▽

Hammer toes **5**

△ Calluses

Dropped metatarsal arch **5**

Crooked big toe **5**

Stand now with your feet parallel, ankles upright, weight evenly distributed, kneecaps facing forward. Lift your toes. Spread them. Place them down on the ground. Now they are alive, working for you. If you stub your toes it hurts a lot. Nature has endowed toes with such acute sensitivity for a purpose. Your toes are in effect your sensors, constantly receiving and transmitting messages — about the ground itself, your relationship with it, your position in space, your balance. And as the roots of a tree serve to anchor it, so your toes are constantly helping to adjust your equilibrium. Toes so often become mere stubby useless appendages. Not only do the feet look less attractive, but the whole being suffers.

The foot is not solid and rigid, but constructed in much the same way as the hand. It has 26 bones articulated by numerous ligaments. There are 12 muscles which span from the lower leg to the foot and another 16 within the foot itself, hence the wonderful dexterity of the foot sometimes achieved by people with no hands. If you walk with a noisy step, or scrape along the ground or clatter up and down stairs, it is probably because you are not using your feet properly. To walk putting the foot down like a flat-iron is a misuse of this amazingly mobile structure, and leads to jarring and lack of grace in the body as a whole. Instead, let your knee float forward so that for a moment your foot drops, hanging loosely, before your heel touches down. As an exercise, you can walk trailing your toes on the ground (as if scuffing the toes of your shoes). Get the feel of the potential suppleness of your feet by walking barefoot, being aware of each segment of the foot as it takes the weight consecutively in a smooth heel-toe action. Above all, be grounded. Sink your weight into your feet. At the same time be centred and let your upper body float upwards, up and out of your waistline.

Walk barefoot as often as you can. An entire therapy, reflexology, is based on massage of points on the foot which are said to relate to organs in the body. This technique is claimed to be both diagnostic and curative. Tender areas on the sole indicate some lack of balance in the corresponding organ. Going barefoot, especially out of doors, over pebbly ground if you can manage it, stimulates all areas of the sole. Not only may this possibly benefit the whole body, it is certain that it strengthens and makes the feet themselves more pliant. It also helps reverse some of the ill effects of wearing unnaturally high heels.

Again, almost every way of sitting on the floor helps stretch tight muscles in the feet and simultaneously gives flexibility to the knees and hips. Sit cross-legged. Kneel back on your heels. Squat. If you can only manage a few seconds in one position, that is enough. Change positions. Change again. You will soon find that it will become more comfortable and that you will be more supple. If you can sit cross-legged easily, sit sometimes with one foot on top of the other leg (remembering to reverse them so that the other foot has its turn on top). If you can kneel back on your heels Japanese-fashion, progress to kneeling between your heels, bottom on the floor. And squat — with your feet parallel, a little way apart, heels on the ground. (Squatting with your heels raised

Norms of Movement

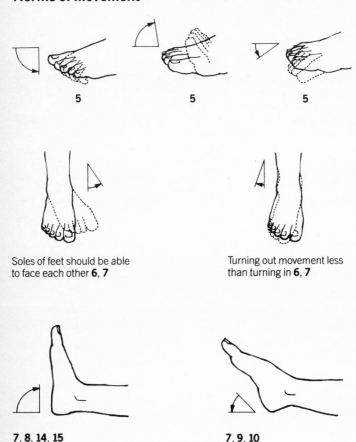

Soles of feet should be able to face each other **6, 7**

Turning out movement less than turning in **6, 7**

7, 8, 14, 15

7, 9, 10

is a strain and will not make you nearly as flexible.) Relax, read, do odd jobs on the floor. You will probably soon prefer it to sitting on a chair.

Finally, never neglect your footwear. Socks, stockings and shoes should leave adequate room for the toes. The thinnest stockings, if they are too tight or too short, can cramp, deform and immobilize your toes. High heels are best kept for the rarest of special occasions. Worn habitually they cause the calf muscles to shorten. Foot movement becomes limited, you become less graceful, and all manner of orthopaedic and gynaecological troubles are encouraged.

The body and the inner state of being both reflect and affect each other. Rigidity of the one is likely to be mirrored in rigidity of the other. Practitioners of the Metamorphic Technique (a type of therapeutic foot massage) suggest, for example, that feet pointing in different directions show confusion, a person who does not know which way she or he is going. Curling toes, hammer toes, bunions, dropped or exaggerated arches, even calluses, corns, chilblains and ingrowing toenails, are each claimed to be significant on a deeper level. Not only will these exercises give you stronger and more flexible feet, you may find that they will influence and improve your whole stance towards your life.

5 Toe Straightener

Strengthens toes and metatarsal arch

Lift your toes. Lift them more. Spread them. Spread them as much as possible. And more.

Now place them down flat. Keeping your heels still, shorten your foot (toes straight, pads pressing into the ground). Hold. Breathe easily. Release. (Repeat.)

Stand with your feet parallel, toes pointing forward and bodyweight divided equally between the heel and ball of your feet. Each toe should be able to lift almost to a right angle (80° is the norm). Aim to lift *all* your toes. Work extra hard on any toes which do not lift. Spread the lifted toes out as far as possible. You should be able to slip a finger simultaneously between each toe. Concentrate on any toes which stay glued together, especially

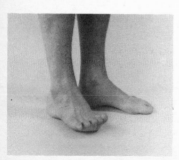
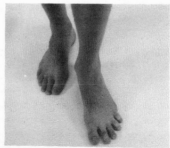

your little toe and your big toe. Place them down flat, straightening them more with your fingers if need be. Now shorten your foot by dragging the pads of the toes back on the ground towards your heel. To do this you need to lift from the little knuckles which lie hidden behind your toes. Concentrate on the four outer toes, keeping them straight as you shorten. It is a tiny caterpillar-like action, the reverse of picking up a pencil with your toes. The toes do not curl under but remain straight or even bend backwards. The knuckles become quite prominent just like those in the hand. (Note that the big toe is unable to perform quite this action as, like the thumb, it is jointed in one place instead of two and has no 'lumbrical' muscle which produces movement in the other toes. It does, however, *bend* at its junction with the forefoot, so it can join in the action, though the emphasis remains with the four outer toes.)

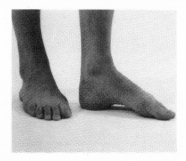

The Benefit
The *lifting* straightens and strengthens the toes. It helps counteract any tendency for them to curl under. The *parting* helps strengthen the front of the foot and also helps improve the structure and alignment of the whole foot. Bunions, dropped metatarsal arches, hammer toes (toes which bend up at the first joint, instead of lying flat) can all result from weak toe-parting muscles. The *shortening* helps straighten the four small toes, strengthen the metatarsal arch and alleviate metatarsal pain in the ball of the foot. It can help to overcome callosities — both the big callus which sometimes develops under the ball of the foot as nature's way of shoring up the structure when the arch is weak, and the ugly little calluses which sometimes develop on top of hammer toes in a vain attempt to act as a buffer between the out-of-place joints and the shoes.

Cautions

1 Exercise sandals, the ones with shaped wooden soles and a ridge under the toes, only strengthen the feet if you use this 'lumbrical' or caterpillar action. They defeat their own purpose if you keep them on, as most people do, by curling the toes.

2 Never pick up pencils with your toes unless you have perfectly straight toes. This will only increase their tendency to curl.

6 Feet In/Feet Out

Strengthens and loosens foot

Sit on the floor, legs outstretched. Point your toes. Turn the soles in to face each other. Turn them in more. Hold. Breathe easily.

Then turn the feet away from each other. Keep on turning until they are pulled right up. Turn still more. And hold. Release. (Repeat.)

Aim for as big a movement as possible from the turned-in position to the turned-out position. This is not an ankle movement. Only the fronts of the feet turn. Do not allow the ankles or knees to roll from side to side. The aim is *mobility* of the feet, *stability* of the legs. The feet move independently of the legs and ankles.

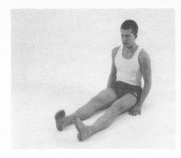 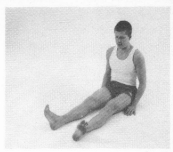

The Benefit
Whenever you walk over rough ground you need the flexibility of
this in-and-out movement. Your feet then adapt to the uneven
surface and act as shock-absorbers. Without this mobility the leg
takes the impact, instead of the foot, and every step can cause
jarring and strain of knees, hips and indeed the whole body. You
should be able to walk over uneven ground as easily as on the flat.

7 Feet Down/Feet Up

**Strengthens and loosens ankle,
strengthens and stretches calf**

*Sit on the floor, legs outstretched. Point your toes. Point them
more. Then pull them up. And more. Breathe easily.* (Repeat.)

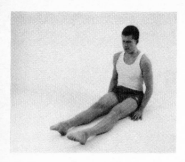 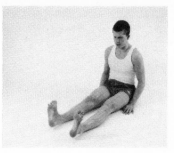

Stretch your feet down to form a straight line, or better still a gentle curve, from the tops of your knees to the tips of your toes. Then pull them up as far as you can keeping them straight (both sides pulled up equally, soles facing directly forwards and not turning in). Do it both very slowly and as quickly as possible. You should be able to pull up to a right angle — 90° — and point down to at least 45°. Anything less is restricted. Aim for a ballet-dancer point, and when you pull up think of the upturned feet of a Balinese dancer.

The Benefit
A smooth graceful walk necessitates a free heel-toe action; the negotiation of hills and stairs depends on it. The whole body moves in an ungainly way if the ankles are stiff. Pointing and pulling up help loosen and strengthen them. Performed slowly, pointing strengthens the deep calf muscle, the muscle of stability. Done quickly, the superficial rounded bulk of the calf, the muscle of speed, is strengthened.

Note
If you are in the habit of wearing high heels, pull your feet up (and do The Lunge and Squatting, nos. 8 and 15) whenever you remember, as they will all help counteract some of the inevitable muscle shortening.

8 The Lunge

Stretches calf and front of hip

Stand in a stride position with one foot in front of the other, both feet facing forward. Bend your front knee, weight over the front foot. Push your back knee hard back. Press your back heel into the ground. And more. Breathe easily. Hold. Release. (Repeat with alternate legs.)

Make sure your feet are in line, toes facing directly forward. Keep your back foot straight, your back heel rooted to the ground, your bottom in and your back flat. This exercise works on the *back* leg, stretching muscles which are too tight in the back of the calf and the front of the hip. You will lose the effect of the stretch if your back foot turns out, your heel lifts off the ground, your bottom sticks out or your back hollows. Look at your back foot. Straighten it if need be so that it is in line with the other one. It should be almost behind the other foot as in a normal stride, not splayed out to the side. Press your hip forward to avoid any sagging at the front. Keep your spine as flat and unhollowed as possible. Make sure your hips and shoulders are square to the front and not turning to the side. The size of the stride is determined by your present degree of flexibility. Take as long a step as possible whilst keeping your heel on the ground. Start with a small step and gradually increase it as you loosen up. Tight calf muscles will quickly surrender to a little daily attention. You will soon find that you can take a much larger stride.

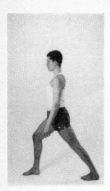
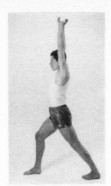

Once you have mastered the simple Lunge and are able to balance comfortably with a long stride, heel down and knee back, you can convert the movement into a satisfying all-over body stretch. Breathing easily, in the lunge position, take your arms out to the side, and over your head. Link your fingers, turn your palms up to the sky. Pull your arms well back, keeping your shoulders low. But remember the primary aim is still the stretch on the *calf*. Even more important now — because it is more difficult with your arms up — keep your back as straight and unarched as you can.

The Benefit
The Lunge stretches muscles in the back of the calf which are often chronically shortened, thus restricting mobility in the foot and fluidity of motion. In women accustomed to wearing high heels the shortening of the calf muscles can become severe. This Lunge does not look as graceful as a fencer's or a dancer's lunge where the back foot turns out, but by releasing shortened calf muscles — which is possible only with the foot straight — you will automatically become more graceful and flowing in your everyday life. This exercise also stretches muscles in the front of the hip which if tight will impose mechanical strain on the body. If shortened on both sides the back will probably be hollow. If shortened on one side only, the leg on that side may be held habitually forward and out to the side, with the foot and knee pointing out.

Caution
Omit this exercise if your ankle is weak or wobbly, as the tight structures (calf muscles and Achilles tendon) may be vital in helping to maintain such stability as there is. To stretch them could render the ankle weaker than ever.

9 Balancing on Tiptoes

Strengthens calf

Stand normally. Lift one foot. Tuck it behind the other leg. Rise on to the tips of the toes of the standing foot. Hover there. Breathe easily. Slowly lower. (Repeat with alternate legs.)

Rise on to the very tips of the toes, pushing your ankle forward so that the front of your foot and leg are in a straight line forming a right-angle with your toes. Aim to pause there. Lower very slowly. (If your balance is shaky, gaze at one point directly ahead and 'centre' yourself.) Normal strength should enable you to do at least six slow lifts without touching the ground with the other foot. When you can do six lifts, do another six. If it is impossible for you to balance on one foot, walk around on tiptoe as a

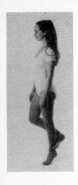

preliminary strengthening measure. Then rise on to the toes of *both* feet and aim to hover there a while. If necessary, hold lightly on to some solid support at first. Gradually it will become easier and you can progress to standing stock still like a stork on just one leg. Finally, close your eyes. It is more difficult now as your balancing mechanisms have to work much harder.

The Benefit
Standing on tiptoe strengthens the calf muscles, especially the deep-lying calf muscle, thus helping balance, stability and body alignment. (The deep calf muscle stabilizes the ankle in standing. If weak it can lead to poor balance and to the bodyweight's being taken over the toes with a forward lean of the whole body, or alternatively to a bent-knee stance.) These are *your* muscles, and they should be capable of supporting (on tiptoes) your own weight, whatever that weight is. Once this is easy, practising with closed eyes is superb balance training.

Note
To exercise the calf thoroughly it is necessary to do rapid movements such as the next, bouncing, exercise, as well as slow movement such as here. There are two types of skeletal muscle fibre in the body. One requires slow movement to strengthen it and the other quick movements. The calf has two large muscles, one composed predominantly of the 'slow' fibres, the other of the 'fast', so for the calf both types of exercise are necessary.

10 Bouncing

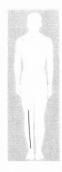

Strengthens calf

*With bare feet, step on the bouncer. Jump up and down —
silently. Breathe easily.*

You need a 'rebounder' or 'bouncer', a sort of mini-trampoline
looking something like a small round coffee table. It is a simple
piece of equipment but a marvellous investment for health and
fitness. Skipping is the time-honoured way of bouncing, but a
bouncer is much more fun. Use your whole foot. Push off with
your toes and point them when you are in mid-air. Land
smoothly, letting your knees 'give' so the jumps are soft and
soundless and there is no jarring. Make sure you do not throw
your head back to gain momentum. Rather keep your neck long
and straight at the back and your chin level. Enjoy yourself.
Choose a lively record and jump to the music.

The Benefit
Firstly, bouncing strengthens the calf muscles, particularly the
superficial muscle which forms the rounded bulk of the calf and
which is the main muscle of propulsion (frogs have a big one). In
athletics it is the muscle of running and jumping, and in everyday
life it helps impart spring and vitality to your walk. It is often
underused and therefore frequently weak, which can result in
hyperextended knees, a not-infrequent postural fault in which the
legs are bowed backwards. This muscle needs rapid movement to

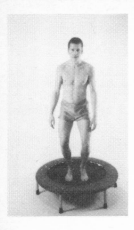 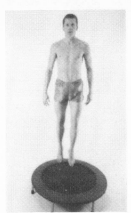

strengthen it. Maximum strengthening is gained by pointing the toes hard.

Bouncing also provides one of the finest forms of aerobic exercise. The United States track and field event team used rebound aerobics (bouncing on a bouncer) in their training programme for the 1984 Olympics. It is probably the most concentrated form of aeorobic exercise there is. This means more benefit can be gained quicker. All aerobic exercise is not equal. Rebounding is more concentrated than skipping. Skipping is more concentrated than jogging, jogging more than cycling, cycling more than hard walking and so on. Ten minutes of skipping is supposed to be equivalent to thirty minutes of jogging. The time would be reduced again for rebounding.

The rebounder acts as a shock-absorber, so unlike many other forms of aerobics it gives rise to virtually no jarring of the skeletal system and therefore to none of the foot, ankle and spinal injuries to which joggers, for example, fall prey. In fact, in the United States rebounding has been used successfully for maintaining fitness in injured people and for improving it in people with rheumatoid and osteoarthritis. One could go on. Claims are made that because of the rhythmic gravitational changes — from pure weightlessness like an astronaut in space at the height of the bounce to three times the normal G-force on earth at touch-down — every cell in the body is stimulated and detoxified, improving the texture of the skin, lessening cellulite, increasing energy levels and making the body look younger and feel better. Whatever else, though, it is simple, it is fun, and it is good for you.

Caution
Bouncing is an aerobic exercise. It has a general all-over effect on your system, so it is important to listen to your body and work within your own limits. Never push yourself beyond your limits, and never allow anybody else to push you.

Note
To exercise the calf thoroughly, it is necessary to do some slow, sustained movement such as the previous exercise, Balancing on Tiptoes, as well as rapid movement such as here.

ADVICE FOR THIGHS

(Knee, front thigh, back thigh)

For the knees to function optimally, to remain trouble-free throughout life and to look as good as knees should look, many of the factors discussed in the previous chapter on the feet are critical. If your toes or kneecaps do not point directly forward and if your bodyweight is not taken evenly, there will be an imbalance of the muscles and ligaments which support the knee. Some will inevitably shorten; those on the other side of the knee will become lax; pockets of fat may collect. The structure is weakened. Strain may then be referred into the hip and possibly into the back. So make sure your feet are straight, that your kneecaps do not squint and that your ankles do not roll in or bow out.

Sitting on the floor is as beneficial for the knees as it is for the feet and ankles. Nothing will help you more to retain – or regain – your youthful spring. When you stand up do not help with your hands, but use the muscles of your legs instead. It may take a little practice at first, but once mastered it need never be lost.

The Ideal

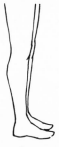

Kneecaps facing forwards   Knees straight

Common Deviations

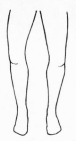

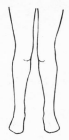

Bowlegs **13**, **16**, **17** (variation 2)

Knock-knees **13**, **16**, **18**, **19**, **23**, **24**

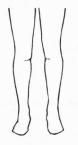

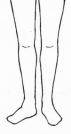

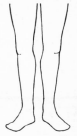

Kneecaps facing in, feet straight **16**, **18**

Kneecaps straight, feet turning out **16**, **18**

Kneecaps and feet turning out **17** (variation 2)

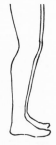

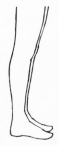

Bent knees **7**, **9**, **14**, **19**, **23**, **24**

Knees curved back **7**, **8**, **10**, **12**, **13**, **14**, **15**

Norms of Movement

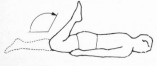

12, 13, 16

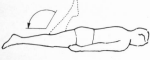

11, 14, 15, 24

Sitting on the floor and standing up unaided by your hands promotes agility and prevents or overcomes much of the rigidity associated with increasing age.

Graceful knees are straight but relaxed. They should not be permanently bent, nor should they be hyperextended (locked tight in a backward curve). Both are signs of weakness and indicate mechanical strain. In the standing position they should be quite straight or extended back only a very few degrees beyond the vertical. If your knees curve back, release them. 'Unlock' them. If they are bent and simply refuse to straighten, practice the exercises which lengthen the back of the leg, such as the Leg Stretch (no.14). Balancing on Tiptoes (no.9) may also help. Miracles of gracefulness can be achieved just by the simple expedient of turning your attention to the backs of your knees. A jerky walk becomes smooth, elegant, free. Suddenly you feel loose-limbed, panther-like.

Knock-knees and bowlegs are often only apparent, rather than a structural bony deformity. The fault lies with posture, and can be corrected easily. 'Postural knock-knees' can occur when the knees are hyperextended, with the kneecaps rolling in. This fault is usually accompanied by apparent (again, postural not structural) flat feet. 'Postural bowlegs', on the other hand, can be the result of hyperextended knees with out-facing kneecaps. The arches may then be excessively high, with the bodyweight falling on the outer borders of the feet. In both cases, check that your feet are parallel. 'Unlock' your knees and swivel your thighs until your kneecaps face forward.

If a knee gives way, or lets you down, as a result of injury, disease or for any other reason, do the Knee Brace (no.11) repeatedly. You cannot fail to see results. If your knees are merely stiff, work at the Knee Bend (no.13). Sit on the floor. Bend your knees in any way possible as long as you do not force pain *within* the knee joint. If you own a rocking chair, this can be a great help (and will also benefit anyone who is suffering from arthritis or is otherwise immobilized). The soft, rhythmic motion flexes and extends knees and hips, stimulating the knees' own lubricant, the synovial fluid, and gently easing them into greater mobility.

If your knees are stiff or weak, no matter what the reason, take heart. The biggest muscles in the body support and move the knee, and the bigger the muscle the more rapidly it responds, as a general rule, to the work placed on it. Knees quickly benefit from the very specific exercises which follow. The knee braces strengthen and the knee bends make you more supple. Even if you have no knee problems and your knees never let you down, these simple movements, in firming the front and back of the thigh, will still have an important aesthetic effect.

11 Knee Brace

Strengthens front of thigh

Sit on the floor, legs outstretched, or lie on your back. Pull your toes up. Push your heels away. Brace your knees back. Pull your kneecaps up. Pull – push – brace – pull. Harder. Hold for six seconds. Breathe easily. Release. (Repeat.)

Sit up out of your waistline with your back straight and hands loose – not behind you propping you up. Sit on your sitting bones and not back on your tailbone. Ease your buttocks back. Rock from side to side. You will soon know if you are on your sitting bones. (To keep a trim figure, remember these bones whenever you are in a chair. Only when you are sitting in the right way can your back support itself. When your back is not supporting itself you are encouraging your waist to thicken.) Pull your toes

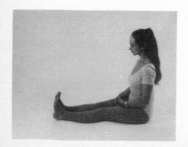

towards you as much as possible, simultaneously pushing your heels hard away. At the same time brace your knees back into the ground and pull your kneecaps up (towards the groin). Concentrate on each element of the knee brace, toes – heels – knees – kneecaps. As you pull your feet to a right-angle keep them straight, soles forward, not turning in. If you brace really hard, your heels will probably leave the ground. When you release, release completely.

Six seconds is about the optimum hold for the purposes of strengthening in a muscle contraction of this type, an isometric contraction. Longer and you could be impeding the circulation, less and the effect is somewhat minimized. Six seconds is quite a long time. To calculate, count 'a-hundred-and-one, a-hundred-and-two' up to 'a-hundred-and-six' (or 'one-cream-cracker, two-cream-cracker . . .' as your fancy takes you). You soon get the feeling of how long to hold without counting. Most important of all in any isometric muscle-hold – or indeed in any sustained activity in daily life – is your breathing. Do not hold your breath. Allow a normal breathing rhythm, always permitting the outbreath. Hanging on to the air can raise your blood pressure and make you tired and stiff the next day.

The Benefit
Simple though it may seem, this is a most powerful means of strengthening. Done slowly, correctly and repetitively, the bracing back of the knee combined with the pulling up of the foot is the basis, the essence, of every effective knee-strengthening technique ever devised, no matter how sophisticated the equipment used. It is specific for the knee that gives way or lets you down. If you are having difficulty in negotiating stairs or hills or in getting up from, or down into, a sitting position, or if you feel any lack of stability in your knees, you cannot do this exercise too often. Bracing can also help straighten those knees which are locked in a backward curve, and work miracles in firming up the fronts of flabby thighs.

12 Kneeling Lie-Back

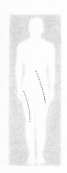

Stretches front of thigh and hip

Kneel back on your heels, then sit between them, bottom on the ground. Lean back supporting yourself on your forearms. Slide your arms forward, gently lowering yourself back to a lying position. Relax into the position. Hold. Breathe easily. Release. (Repeat.)

Take the whole movement very gently, only doing what you can do, little by little, day by day. Do not force anything. Kneel back on your heels. If it is difficult, take some weight on your hands, easing yourself down a little further each time you breathe out. A strong pull on the fronts of the feet, ankles or thighs indicates muscle shortening. Allow the stretch. It is entirely beneficial, and with a little practice the tension will soon be released. However,

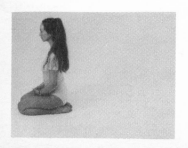 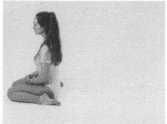

avoid pain *within* the knee joint. Only when it is comfortable to kneel *on* the heels should you proceed to the next stage, kneeling *between* them. Again use your hands to help you, if you need to. When kneeling between your heels is comfortable, but only then, lean back taking your bodyweight on your forearms. At this point hitch your bottom forward. Finally ease yourself right back, keeping your chin on your chest until the last moment. Once down, place your head carefully so that it rests on the base, not the top, of your skull. Allow your upper back to settle into the floor. Then turn your attention to your lower back. It is most unlikely to touch the ground, but allow it to drop as much as you can. The flatter it is the more you will stretch the front of your hips and the greater the benefit you will derive from the exercise. Breathe easily, and with each outbreath let go of any straining – or arching – in the back and neck. Finally, when this position has

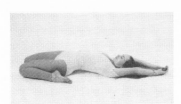

become quite comfortable, you can stretch your arms above your head, aiming eventually to lay them flat on the ground.

The Benefit
Overtaut foot, ankle, thigh and hip muscles at the front are stretched and relaxed. This promotes greater flexibility in the whole leg and allows better alignment at the hip between leg and body. The stretch on the hip muscle helps counteract a hollow back and the mechanical strain on the body that that induces. Walking becomes more fluid and movement more graceful.

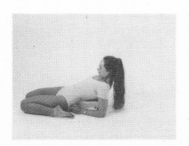
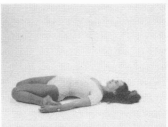

Finally, a marvellous whole-body stretch is produced by taking the arms back over the head. It is a wonderfully invigorating exercise.

Cautions
1 Omit this exercise if it causes pain *within* the knee joint, as it may be aggravating problems there.
2 Avoid kneeling back on your heels if you have varicose veins.
3 Be careful when you are kneeling between your heels to rest on the tops and not the inner borders of your feet. If you twist your feet, you may strain the feet or knees.
4 Do not kneel on your heels too often if you habitually wear high heels as it can reinforce the specific muscle imbalance likely to be present.

13 Knee Bend

Strengthens back of thigh, stretches front of thigh

Lie on your front. Keeping your thigh down, bend one knee, heel to buttock. Bend hard. Breathe easily.

Continuing to bend, lift your thigh. More. Release. (Repeat with alternate legs.)

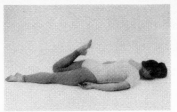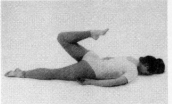

The whole body should be easy and relaxed. Let your hip sink into the ground to anchor you well down. Do not be tempted to lift it and to roll your body to gain extra movement. Aim to touch your bottom. If you have less than 130° bend your knees are stiff. There are two distinct actions to this knee bend – thigh down and thigh raised. Extract the maximum from each one.

The Benefit
This exercise increases the flexibility of the knee (especially in the 'thigh down' position) and firms the back of the thigh (especially in the 'thigh raised' position). By strengthening the back-thigh (or hamstring) muscles, the full bend with the thigh raised can also help straighten a hollow back.

Cautions
1 Avoid pain *within* the knee joint itself as this may indicate and aggravate internal knee problems. A strong stretch on the front of the thigh, however, is positive and shows that you can benefit from bending in this way.
2 If your knee is unstable and gives way easily, it is more important to strengthen than to stretch the front-thigh muscles. In this case, build the muscles up with plenty of knee bracing (no.11). Introduce knee bending gradually when the knee is a little stronger.

14 Leg Stretch

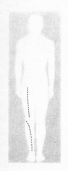

Stretches calf and back of thigh

Lie on your back. Lift one leg. Link your fingers behind your thigh. Brace back your knee. Pull your toes towards you, push your feet away.

Now, keeping your raised leg firm, lift your head and shoulders and slide your hands towards your foot. Breathing easily, your leg remaining firm, slowly let your back drop to the ground. Bring your leg closer still, sliding your hands even nearer to your foot. (Repeat with alternate legs.)

The raised leg stays firm, knee braced back, toes towards you throughout. The other leg lies flat on the ground and does not bend. On each exhalation brace the leg further. Keep your shoulders relaxed as you lift your head to creep your hands up

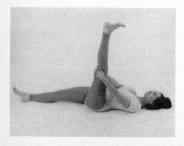

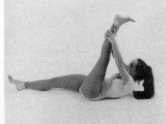

your leg. Then very very slowly indeed, chin on chest, allow your back to drop towards the ground. Let your lower back touch down first, then your upper back and shoulders, then the base of your skull. Take as much time as you wish. There is no effort, no force. Gravity does the work in its own slow time. Finally – and only when you are comfortably on your back – bring your leg as close to your body as you can, still bracing your knee and sliding your hands even further towards your feet.

The Benefit

If you cannot reach very far up your leg this is *not* (tall people) because your legs are too long or (small people) because your arms are too short, it is because your back-thigh muscles, your hamstrings, are too tight. Your muscles should be able to relax sufficiently to permit you to reach well up. With comparatively little practice, they will. Allowing your back to drop down in this way, and eventually pulling the leg closer to the body, helps restore normal length to the hamstring muscles. When they are tight – shortened – they exert an abnormal pull on the knees and pelvis, encouraging bent knees and reduced, less-than-normal curves of the low back. (If the low back is too flat, the hamstring muscles should always be checked.) Finally, pushing your heel away stretches the calf and helps loosen the ankle. There are many ways of stretching your hamstrings – touching the toes is one – but there can be a danger of hurting the back. This is a particularly safe way, as the low back is supported and the muscles 'give' slowly in their own time.

Cautions

1 Go easy on this exercise at first if you have a bad back, or omit it altogether if you think your back will not take it. On no account cause pain in your low back as you can damage yourself. A

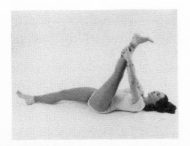

pulling in the back of the leg, however, indicates that the muscles are crying out to be stretched.

2 Whilst shortened hamstring muscles reduce the normal curve of the spine, lax hamstrings can lead to a hollow back and associated weakness of the abdominal muscles. This can sometimes be clearly seen in highkicking dancers. They can kick their legs high, unrestricted by tight back-thigh muscles, but their backs are chronically overarched. (The same sway-back can result from yoga practised thoughtlessly.) Both flat back and hollow back are the legacy of muscle imbalance. The normal length of the hamstrings is such that, lying on your back, your legs can be lifted passively (i.e. by someone else), one leg at a time, to an 80° or 85° angle from the ground without having to bend the other leg or arch the back. Over 90° is regarded as excessive. So the position is simple. Loosen up until you can achieve the anatomical norm of 85°. If you have a hollow back, do not attempt to stretch further. If or when you can lie on your back with the small of the back sinking quite naturally into the floor without any strain whatsoever you can safely stretch the hamstrings as much as you wish.

3 'Back knees', legs which bow back at the knee, are often the result of lax hamstring muscles and it is unwise to stretch them further until normal strength and alignment are regained. Use the Knee Bend (no.13) and the Leg Backward Lift (no.16) to strengthen them, and always stand with your knees slightly relaxed rather than locked back.

15 Squatting

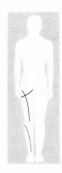

Strengthens front of thigh and buttock, stretches calf

Stand with your feet parallel and a little way apart, toes facing forward. Keeping your heels on the floor, gently lower yourself to a squat. Breathe easily. Hold. Stand up. (Repeat.)

Check that your feet and knees are straight, pointing directly ahead so that your knees are able to bend *forward* over your feet. Keeping your heels on the ground, sit back on your haunches. Do not strain by sticking your bottom up. Imagine instead that you have a weight at the end of your spine pulling your tailbone down. Your back will now be gently rounded, not ramrod

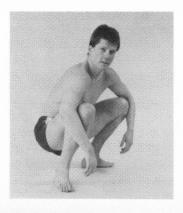

straight. Let your bodyweight fall centrally over your feet and not too much over the inner borders or the heels. Are your feet still parallel? They should be. Look straight ahead, not up in the air or down at the ground. The important thing is to keep your heels down. If it is difficult to squat without raising your heels, simply bend as far as you can, heels on the ground. Quietly observe your breathing for a moment then dip down a little further on each outbreath. You will derive much more benefit from squatting just a little way with your heels down than by doing a full knees-bend with heels raised. As this is very much a natural movement, surprisingly little practice is usually required to drop right down in the squat. After a moment, stand up as slowly as you can. If squatting with the heels down is easy, relax in the position sometimes instead of sitting in a chair. It is immensely beneficial. Put your hands on your head to make it more difficult. Then bend down and stand up on *one* leg. Not so easy!

The Benefit
Standing up from the squat is very good for strengthening and firming the front-thigh and buttock muscles, as they must work to raise the whole weight of the body against gravity. Squatting itself, and lowering oneself into the squat, are potent aids to flexibility of the ankle, knee and hip joints. Squatting also helps to stretch the deep calf muscle which is often shortened owing to the unnatural practices of 'civilized' living – chairs, plumbing facilities which take no account of human anatomy, fashionable if orthopaedically disastrous high-heeled shoes. If shortened, the knees may be bowed backwards in standing and the toes turned out in walking. (If you do wear high heels a lot, squatting is especially important to help counteract the imbalance.) As a bonus, many people find squatting helps relieve or prevent constipation.

Cautions
1 Do not force pain *within* the knee joint. This may indicate or aggravate internal knee dysfunction.
2 As always, the aim must be equilibrium. Occasionally, instead of giving a necessary stretch to the calf muscles, repeated squatting can lead to over-stretching and weakness. If you can do the Balancing on Tiptoes (no.9) there is no problem. If not, make sure that you do not favour the one ability at the expense of the other. Aim to develop each (squatting and standing on tiptoes) in balance with the other.

Note

Squatting is a position adopted naturally by small children at play. It should *never* be discouraged in favour of infant-sized chairs, as it promotes normal development of the pelvis, especially important in girls. Chairs, however well designed, do *not* aid normal development in the growing child.

TIPS FOR HIPS

(Hip, outside thigh, inside thigh, buttock)

First of all, check once again that your bodyweight is evenly distributed, feet parallel, kneecaps facing forward. Where the feet and knees are not straight but, in the standing position, point in or out, there is inevitably an associated twist on the thigh. The whole leg is rotated from the hip joint, putting strain on the joint and causing the sort of wear and tear that can lead to osteoarthritis. And as the body is a unity and not simply a series of segments, strain is often referred into the back, putting the whole body at a mechanical disadvantage.

Sitting on the floor is not only excellent for the whole leg but also for the hip and indeed for the spine, as in this position the back has to support itself. Sitting crosslegged on the floor is particularly helpful in keeping the hips mobile and overcoming

The Ideal

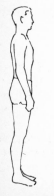 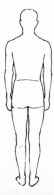

Common Deviations

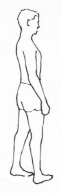

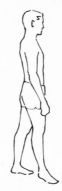

One leg held forward
and turned in **18**

One leg held forward
and turned out **8**, **12**

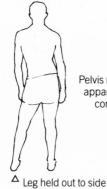

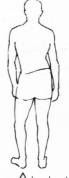

Pelvis raised on one side causing
apparent short leg — other leg
compensates **19**, **23**, **24**

△ Leg held out to side

△ Leg bent

the tendency of the inner thigh muscles, the hip adductors, to shorten. Crossing your legs on a chair, on the other hand, encourages the adductors to tighten up. In addition, it constricts the circulation and is especially to be avoided if there is any suggestion of varicose veins. And, more subtly, it gives the wrong messages about you. It conveys tension; it makes you appear closed, cold, calculating. Crossed legs and folded arms are defensive gestures, protecting the individual but making others feel ill-at-ease in your company.

Norms of Movement

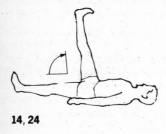

14, **24**

12, **15** (standing up from the squat), **16**, **18**

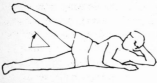

17, **19**, **23**, **24**

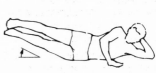

17 (variation 1), **27**

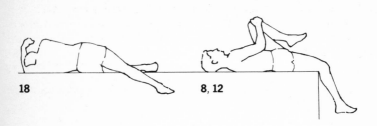

18

8, **12**

The hip is the point at which the legs meet the body, but in another sense our legs are much longer than this. The muscle which takes the leg forward when we walk is attached below to the thigh bone but, at its uppermost point, to the vertebra to which the lowest rib is joined. To find the point, trace your bottom rib round to your backbone. Functionally your leg starts from here – half-way up your back, in fact. For a lithe loose-limbed gait, visualize your leg being drawn forward from the middle of your back. Simultaneously, let your knee float forward and your foot hang loosely in mid-stride before placing your heel down. This gives a smooth, gentle, easy gliding action with the minimum expenditure of energy and exertion.

The buttock muscle is the largest of the hip muscles. If it is tensed up, walking will be more ungainly than it need be. Many people clench their buttocks as an automatic reaction to stress, to difficulty, to embarrassment, in the same way as others hunch their shoulders. Some people keep them constantly clenched. This causes the buttock muscle to overwork, and often enlarges it in quite an ugly way. An enormous amount of energy is expended just in maintaining the tension – energy which should be free-flowing and not locked up. Tensing the body has the power to reduce anxiety, but unfortunately it also shuts off joyful feelings and pleasurable states. Specifically in this area of the pelvis we can deaden ourselves sexually. Tension becomes a kind of protective armour, a denial of growth, learning and expansion. So relax your buttocks. Relax them especially if you think your bottom is too big, or that you do not move attractively, or if you feel you are not getting too much out of sex. Check, when the next awkward moment comes along, that you have not tightened up. If you find that you have, don't worry. Now you can do something about it.

The exercises in this section will help balance the muscles which stabilize your hip, muscles which are vital for your alignment and agility.

16 Leg Backward Lift

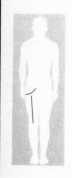

Strengthens buttock and back of thigh

Lie on your front, both legs stretched back. Lift one leg, keeping your hip bone down. Breathe easily. Lift more.

Rotate your leg, heel in – toes out. And more. Hold. Rotate the other way, heel out – toes in.

Slowly turn your heel, in – out – in – out. Lower. (Repeat with alternate legs.)

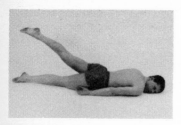

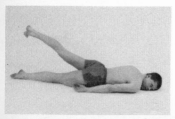

To avoid straining your neck when lying on your front, rest your head on the side of your face or on your forehead, not on your chin. Stretch your legs out, making them as long as you can. When you lift your leg, take care to sink the hip bone into the ground. This limits the actual amount of lift but isolates the back-thigh and buttock muscles (the muscles should be strong enough to raise the leg to an angle of about 15° from the ground).

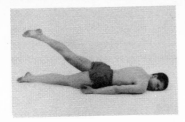

The leg will apparently lift much higher when the hip is not anchored down, but the firming action is lost. Make sure you rotate your leg slowly, turning as much as you can. Throughout the exercise, your arms should be passive and the rest of your body relaxed and at ease. Use your breathing to help you, lifting on the inbreath, sustaining on the outbreath.

The Benefit
This lift strengthens and firms the buttock and back-thigh muscles which are important in the alignment of leg, hip, pelvis and back and which should always be checked, and strengthened if necessary, in low back problems. A weak buttock muscle makes it difficult to get up from a sitting position without pushing up with your hands, besides ensuring a sagging backside and leaving you stiff, ungainly, heavy and uncoordinated. Weak back-thigh (hamstring) muscles in both legs predispose towards a hollow back. Weak hamstrings in one leg allow the pelvis to twist forward on the weak side. If the inner hamstrings are weak, the inside of the knee loses its stability and there is a tendency to knock-knees. Outer hamstring weakness predisposes towards bowlegs. All these kinds of imbalance and strain can be helped by the differing rotations in this lift.

17 Leg Sideways Lift

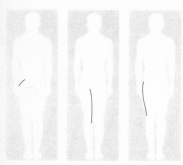

Strengthens side of hip

Variation 1   Variation 2

Lie on one side comfortably balanced, lower leg bent, upper leg in line with the body. Lift your upper leg as high as you can, keeping your foot parallel with the ground. Breathe easily. Lift higher. Hold. And lift more. Slowly lower. (Repeat with alternate legs.)

Make sure you are well supported on your side and not rolling over backwards. You can cradle your head in your arms for support. The lower leg is bent, not only for comfort, but because it allows the upper leg to drop further down, increasing the range of the lift and, correspondingly, the strengthening effect. Three points are important. First, make sure the upper leg is in line with the body. This generally means having it much further back than one expects. There should be no forward angle at the hip but a

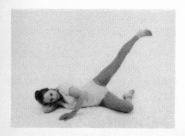

strong backward stretch. Secondly, the leg must be 'lengthened' before and during the lift so that it is not retracted into the hip. Thirdly, the lower border of the foot should remain parallel with the floor during the lift. If the heel drops the hip will rotate outwards and the strengthening effect of the movement is largely lost. Done the wrong way – leg forward and shortened, heel down and toes up – you can produce a magnificent lift. Anyone can. But it will be useless. With the leg back and 'long' the lift will be much less – about 45° from the ground is the norm – but you will be strengthening one of the most important muscles of the body.

The Benefit
This exercise strengthens the main outer hip muscle, one of the key muscles of the body which affects alignment, stability and gracefulness. This muscle lifts the leg out to the side away from the body and stabilizes the leg at the hip. Often it is weak on one side as a result of the lop-sided right- or left-handed way we use our bodies (the right muscle is often weak, strangely, in right-handed people and the left, though less consistently, in left-handed people). The results are far-reaching. Right-sided weakness, for example, leads to the pelvis being high and the shoulder low on the right, with a resultant sideways spinal curvature, a 'C' curve, convex to the left. This in mild degree is very common indeed. Severe weakness on one side produces a characteristic lurching gait which at worst can become a pronounced limp. Weakness on both sides produces a waddle. If, however, the outer hip muscle is strong, even if many of the numerous other muscles acting on the hip are injured or weak, it is possible to walk, even run, with amazingly little disability. This simple exercise, done on one or both sides, as appropriate, can have a near-transforming effect on appearance and coordination.

Variation I – Inside-Thigh Strengthener

Lie on your side with both legs straight. Lift your upper leg about 25° from the ground. Bring the lower leg up to join it. Hold. Breathe easily. Slowly lower. This helps firm up the inside thigh of the underneath leg. (See also Waistline Firmer, no.27.)

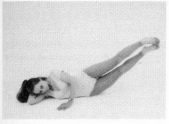

Variation I

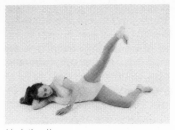

Variation II

Variation II – Outside-Thigh Strengthener

This helps if there is a tendency to bowlegs with the feet turning out when standing. Again, lie on your side with your legs straight. Keep the lifting leg 'long' and the lower border of the foot parallel with the ground as before, but have the leg at an angle of 45° *in front* of the body instead of in line with it. When the leg is as high as you can lift it – 30° is the norm – turn the foot so the heel is up and the toes are pointing down. Hold. Breathe easily. Lift a little higher, then slowly lower.

18 Kneeling Crossover

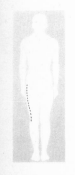

Stretches outside thigh

Kneel. Cross one leg over and behind the other, lower legs and feet parallel and resting on the ground. Hold. Breathe easily. (Repeat on alternate sides.)

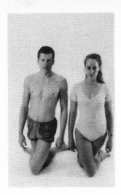 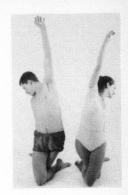

Your hips should face directly ahead – swivel them forwards if necessary. Make sure your back is straight and your chin level. When you can hold this position quite easily for a few breaths, with your right leg crossed behind your left, lift your right arm above your head. Your elbow should be straight, upper arm against your ear. Swivel your hips further to the left, letting your head and shoulders follow. Breathing easily, aim to touch your left heel with your left hand. Change sides. Repeat.

The Benefit
This exercise helps stretch the outside thigh muscles of the crossing leg. When these are tight there is often a tendency to knock-knees and/or infacing kneecaps combined with a hollow back. If just one outside thigh muscle is short, only the one leg will be affected and instead of a hollow back the pelvis may be low on the tight side. In this case do the exercise on one side only until greater balance is achieved.

19 Splits Stretch

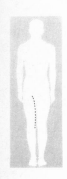

Stretches inside thigh

Sit with your legs outstretched and separated. Separate them still further. And further. Breathe easily. And separate them more.

Roll your feet and knees out. Hold. Release. (Repeat several times.)

Sit up straight, spine vertical. It is not too easy to sit straight with your legs spread, so check yourself before you begin and keep straightening if you slump. Sit on your sitting bones and not back on your tailbone. The aim is simply to part your legs as much as you can (and more), and *then* to roll your knees out. You will probably feel a very powerful – and beneficial – stretch on the

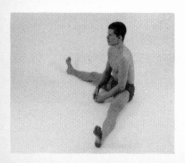

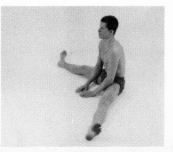

inside thigh. (If not, you are one of the few people who do not need this exercise!) If you cannot form a right-angle, 90°, between the two legs, movement is definitely restricted.

The Benefit
This stretch helps lengthen the muscles of the inner thigh which are often shortened. These muscles act to bring the thighs together and used to be called the 'morality muscles'. In women this shortening is often a direct result of being taught from earliest childhood to sit in a ladylike manner with the legs together. (However, it is not only women who are afflicted with tense morality muscles.) When the inside thigh muscles are shortened, the hips are rigid. This makes it difficult, for example, to sit cross-legged on the ground because the knees stick up awkwardly in the air instead of relaxing down. If the muscles are shortened on one side only the leg itself will probably appear short. Any activity requiring a spreading-out of the legs is also more difficult – for instance, riding on horseback – and it can become harder, as well, to correct knock-knees or a hollow back.

MIDRIFF MATTERS

(Abdomen and back)

The abdomen and back are an entity, two sides of the same coin. Whilst each has its own distinct set of muscles, which can be worked on separately, the total picture is important. A frequent pattern is for the abdominal muscles to be weak and over-stretched (too long) while the corresponding muscles in the low back are too tight (shortened). The result is a bulging abdomen and a sway back, as well as a predisposition to backache. Compensating for an overarched low back there can be a rounding of the upper back and, intimately linked with both, an arching back of the neck with lifted chin and upturned face. The slack upper back muscles may lead to a shortening of the muscles across the chest, with round shoulders and restricted arm movement. (The neck and shoulder are dealt with, for conveni-ence, in their own sections later, but they are an integral part of the pattern.)

Overall, then, there is often a tendency for the spinal curves to become excessive, with the neck and low back concave (muscles too short and tense), the upper back convex (muscles too long and weak) and a loss of length in the spine as a whole. There *should* be curves in the spine, but if they are exaggerated – or, as occasionally happens, reduced – the body is off-balance and under strain. The alignment we have – straight back, hollow back, round back – is not a 'given', but is largely under our own control. It does not arise from the shape of the spine but from the habitual pull of the muscles which attach to it.

Ideally if you lie flat on your back with your legs straight and your head level, your low back should drop of its own accord so there is no space at all between it and the ground. You should then, still on your back but with your legs bent and soles on the ground, be able to curl up, hands behind head, to a sitting position. If this is possible you have nothing to worry about. Simply maintain this 'normal' strength and alignment throughout your life. If not, there is muscular imbalance. This chapter will help you overcome it.

The Ideal

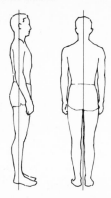

Common Deviations

Exaggerated upper back curve
('kyphosis') **12** (arms above head),
21 (arms above head), **25**, **40**,
41, **42**
Exaggerated lower back curve
('hollow back' or 'lordosis') **4**,
8, **12**, **13**, **16**, **18**, **19**, **20**, **21**, **22**,
23, **24**, **26**, **27**, **28**, **29**

Reduced curve **26** ▷

Reduced curve ▷
('no bottom') **14**, **24**

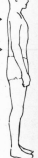

Sideways spinal curvature ('C-curve scoliosis') **12**
(arms above head), **17**, **21** (arms above head),
22, **23**, **24**, **25**, **26**, **27**, **28**, **29**, **40**, **41**, **42**

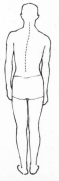

To exercise your back and abdomen safely and to achieve the best results it is helpful to understand a little of their anatomy.

The muscles of the stomach form in effect a four-way reinforced corset extending from the pelvis below to the ribcage above. There are four muscles at either side, a horizontal, a vertical and two diagonal muscles. Together they form a four-way cross, something like a Union Jack. Each of the muscles is attached in the midline to the 'linea alba', the thin dark vertical line which is often visible below the navel but which in fact extends all the way from the pubic bone up to the breast bone. The horizontal and oblique muscles wrap around the waist and into the back so that strengthening them also helps to neaten the waistline and sides, as well as firming the front.

These muscles are sandwiched between two layers of fat. From the outside in, there is the skin, then a layer of fat, then the muscles, then fat, then a lining (the peritoneum), then the intestines and abdominal organs, also padded around with fat. Many people crave to be 'hollow' in front, but this is not healthy, as it indicates tension in the muscles and almost certainly means that the organs are cramped and breathing restricted. The outline, however, should be only very gently rounded and the muscles should be firm. Because they run in different directions, there is no one exercise that optimally strengthens each muscle simultaneously. A balanced selection – for example, the Stomach Lift (no.20), the Pelvic Tilt (no.21) and the Curl-Ups (no.22) – is needed.

Strong abdominal muscles are vital not only to appearance but to general health, alignment and comfort. They protect the abdominal and pelvic organs which, unlike the heart and lungs enclosed in the ribcage, have very little bony protection, and they are designed to maintain the ideal pressure for the functioning of these organs, and to compress them sufficiently to hold them in their ideal position. With the exception of the horizontal muscle, whose sole function is protection and compression, the muscles also act to produce movement. In various combinations they lift the body from a lying position, bend it, and twist it sideways. And they are important in breathing where strong expiratory effort is needed. Normally, no muscular effort is required to breathe out, but in coughing, sneezing, vomiting, elimination, in childbirth, even in singing and shouting, the help of the abdominal muscles is required.

In association with the abdominal musculature is the musculature of the back. Like tramlines at either side of the spine, long

Norms of Movement

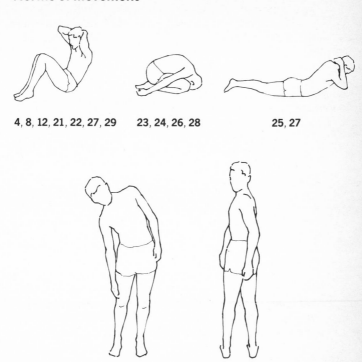

4, 8, 12, 21, 22, 27, 29   23, 24, 26, 28   25, 27

28   22, 27, 29

vertical muscles run from sacrum to skull. They are composite muscles made up of many smaller muscles attaching to the individual vertebrae, and have the vital task of supporting the spine. Usually, they are strong in the low back, but in the upper back they are often weak and elongated. Contrary to popular opinion, however weak or tired or really painful the low back feels, the chances are that strengthening the muscles there is not the answer. They are almost certainly strong already and, especially if the back is hollow, need to be stretched rather than strengthened.

In almost all cases of low back trouble any muscular weakness is likely to be abdominal, and this should be the main focus of attention. The optimum low back curve and the correct tilt of the pelvis is maintained by the upward pull of firm abdominal muscles in front combined with a strong downward pull from the buttock muscles behind. If these muscles are slack, the pelvis tilts, the low back arches too much, and the whole body is thrown out of alignment and put under strain. (The pelvis should also be level from side to side. If the right and left muscles are of unequal strength, a sideways curvature of the spine may result. This can be helped by doing certain exercises on one side only, as indicated in the text.)

Much of the ordinary daily activity of sedentary life – the way we sit, stand, or walk on flat ground – does not put enough demand on the muscles in this part of the body. The exercises in this section are largely designed to strengthen the abdomen, stretch the low back, strengthen the upper back, and increase mobility generally.

Cautions

1 Do *not* do straight-back sit-ups with straight legs. These will only strengthen the front hip (or walking) muscles, which are almost always strong already and often overcontracted. You will be *stretching* your abdomen and buttocks – increasing the flab. Instead, do rounded-back Curl-Ups (no.22).

2 Do *not* anchor your feet under a piece of furniture, or let anyone else hold them down, when you do Curl-Ups. This forces your back into a very vulnerable position which can lead to backache or real back damage.

3 Do *not* raise both legs together straight. You are overstretching the muscles of the pelvic floor, especially inadvisable in women as it can lead to sexual and gynaecological difficulties.

4 Do *not* touch your toes with legs straight. The hamstring muscles, which cross the back of the thigh from pelvis to calf, act to bend the knee and pull the thigh back at the hip. Touching your toes with your knees straight produces the reverse hip and knee action, therefore putting the hamstrings on maximum stretch. The hamstrings are often tight to begin with and tug on the pelvis from below. If, in addition, you have any shortening, rigidity or hollowing of the low back, the back muscles will be tugging at the pelvis from above. You can thus exert an enormous pull from both above and below, so running a high risk of back damage.

20 Stomach Lift

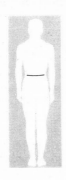

Strengthens abdomen

Stand, knees bent, feet a little way apart. Support yourself, hands on thighs. Exhale as strongly as possible.

Keeping all the air expelled . . . retract your abdomen. Hold it in until you need to inhale. Then gently release and breathe in. (Repeat.)

Support yourself firmly and comfortably, knees bent, arms straight. Your back should be rounded not hollowed (an arched back would merely distend the stomach and interfere with the contraction of the muscle). Breathe out hard, then pull in and up, stomach to backbone. There is a definite feeling of suction within

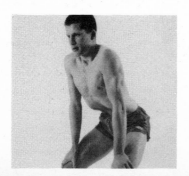

the abdomen when you pull in with the air expelled, quite different from the feeling when you simply tighten your stomach while breathing normally. The abdominal area becomes a hollow basin, its rim the pelvic bones and lower ribcage. The bones are then so prominent that you can grasp them with your hands. When you need to breathe again, slowly release your abdomen and *then* breathe in. The Stomach Lift is self-limiting – your body will tell you when you have had enough.

Common faults when doing the Stomach Lift are either to start pulling the abdomen in before completing the exhalation, or surreptitiously to breathe in a little air as you pull the muscle in. The firming, strengthening effect is then lost. You will know when you are doing it correctly by the sensation of a vacuum within and by your wonderfully concave abdomen. (If you feel a tightening in your throat as you close off the air passages there is no need to worry unless it is too uncomfortable, in which case omit the exercise for the time being.) Once you have mastered the Stomach Lift, see if you can stand up straight, maintaining your flatter-than-flat stomach. (This, of course, is purely an exercise, *not* the way to stand normally.)

The Benefit

The Stomach Lift helps tighten the transverse muscle which wraps around the waist and which is probably the major factor in determining your contour. As this muscle is strengthened and shortened the abdomen in front firms up and the waistline to the sides becomes slimmer and neater. (Signs of its weakness are a sway back, or a sideways bulge when doing Curl-Ups or Back-Bends.) Since the function of the transverse muscle is wholly one of compression and protection, and unlike the other abdominal muscles it does not produce actual movement, there is no corresponding movement by which it can be strengthened. The Stomach Lift, however, does help to tone it and can have a powerful effect on your appearance.

Caution

Strenuous exercises, and particularly abdominal exercises, should not be practised immediately after a meal.

21 Pelvic Tilt

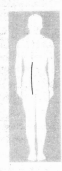

Strengthens abdomen

*Lie on your back. Keeping your legs still and your head level
. . . drop the small of your back to the floor. Hold. Breathe
easily. Push down more. Release.* (Repeat.)

Adjust your head so that it is resting on the back, not the top, of
the skull. The chin should be level, not poking up in the air. The
back of the neck should lie parallel with the floor and the face
parallel with the ceiling. Take care to maintain this position as
you press your low back to the floor. Your head may want to roll
back so that the chin sticks up and the back of the neck arches. In
this case you are merely shunting the hollow from your back up to
your neck. Likewise do not displace any hollowing down to your
legs. If your knees bend when you flatten your back, push your
heels away from you and pull your toes towards you. And
breathe. Breathe *out.* Do nothing to change your breathing.
Simply be aware of the rhythm, always allowing the outbreath.

In an ideal situation, the small of the back should sink naturally

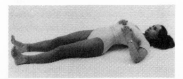
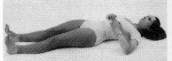

to the floor (the low back does have a natural concave curve, but this should be so slight that when you lie down the weight of the body and the pull of gravity flatten it out completely). Most people, however, find there is a space – often a veritable tunnel – under their back when they lie on the ground. If it is very difficult to drop your back right down without bending your knees or throwing your head back, start with your knees bent and your feet flat on the ground. Your back will then probably touch the floor. If there is still a space, press down as much as you can. Then lift your toes and, keeping your back down, very slowly slide your heels along the ground until your legs are straight. Slide them together or one at a time. If you feel your back or neck arching as you straighten, pause or even bend your knees a fraction more. Drop your back again. Slowly slide your legs down, pausing again to adjust your back if necessary.

The Benefit
The Pelvic Tilt helps strengthen and firm up the vertical band of the abdominal corset. If this muscle is weak there is a tendency towards a hollow back. This exercise strengthens the lower part of the muscle especially, and can have a dramatic effect on the appearance of the lower abdomen, lifting and flattening it. The Curl-Ups (no.22) help strengthen the same muscle, but more particularly the upper part of it. The two exercises can therefore be seen as a unity, between them maximally toning up the whole muscle.

22 Curl-Ups

Strengthens abdomen

Sit on the ground, chin on chest, knees bent, soles flat down, arms loosely by your sides. Slowly curl back to the lying position. Then, keeping your feet still . . . curl up again to the sitting position. Breathe easily.

Now place both hands outside your left knee. Turn to look at your hands. Curl back (on the oblique away from your hands). Curl up again (on the oblique – right elbow to left knee). Breathe easily. Repeat on the other side.

(Repeat in all three directions.)

Both for strengthening the abdominal muscles *and* to protect your back, it is essential to keep your head tucked well forward, your back rounded and your feet on the ground. The key word is 'curl'. These are *not* straight-back sit-ups, which do nothing to strengthen the abdominal muscles. If the back actually arches, the abdominal muscles are in fact overstretched, rather than being shortened and strengthened. So, as you curl down, drop the small of your back then slowly unroll yourself like a carpet. Reverse the procedure as you curl up, keeping your chin on your chest and your low back sinking into the ground until the very last moment. The whole down-and-up curl should be done slowly and smoothly and with perfect control. (If you simply collapse down you achieve nothing but a bruised back. If you throw yourself up

at speed, momentum and not muscle-power does the work.)
Keep your toes on the ground, your legs together and your knees
still, central and stable throughout. Your arms should be passive
– if you use them to help you, your abdominal muscles do
nothing. And, most important of all in such a strong movement,
breathe easily, letting the air come and go.

Always do a set of three curl-ups, a straight one and two
obliques. The straight muscle and the two oblique muscles will
then be strengthened equally and are kept in balance. If one way
is more difficult than the others, do a bit extra in the weak
direction to bring it up to strength. For the oblique movement,

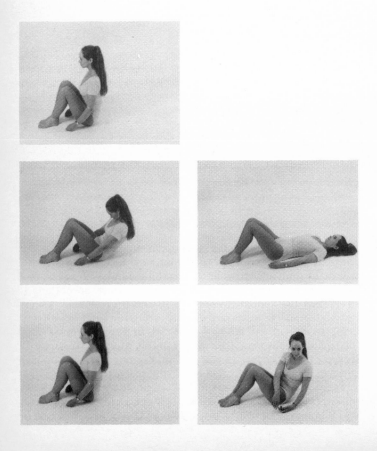

really *turn* your shoulders hard to one side and curl back away from the direction in which you are facing. Curl up again on the oblique to the starting position. Then turn your shoulder hard to the other side and repeat. (Theoretically, only the last part of the downward curl and the first part of the upward curl actually bring the abdominal muscles into play. It is therefore not strictly necessary to come right up to the sitting position, but it makes for a smoother and more satisfying movement if you do.)

When the movement is easy with your arms passively by your sides, progress by changing your hand position. Fold your arms across your chest, placing each hand on the other shoulder (elbow to opposite knee on the oblique movements). If you have to straighten your legs as you come up you are not ready for this hand position yet. When this, too, is easy, clasp your hands behind your head, making sure you keep your elbows well back so they touch the ground as you go down and stay opened out as you come up. Again direct each elbow to the opposite knee on the oblique movements. If you find yourself straightening out your legs as you come up, revert to the previous easier hand position until you are a little stronger. Finally, clasping your hands behind your head, progressively bring your feet closer and closer in, until you can do the Curl-Ups slowly and smoothly with your heels about six inches from your body.

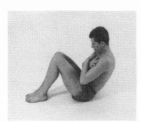 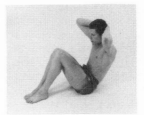

The Benefit
Normal abdominal strength should enable you to curl back and up with your hands behind your head, elbows well back and your feet close to your body. If you cannot do this slowly, easily and with control then your abdominal muscles are weak. Fortunately they are quickly strengthened, and that strength is easily maintained. Like the Pelvic Tilt (no.21), the *straight* Curl-Up primarily helps to strengthen and tighten the vertical band of the abdominal corset. The Curl-Ups help particularly in firming the

upper part of the muscle. (The lower part is helped more by the Pelvic Tilt.) It is this vertical muscle which bends the spine forward, providing the movement is against gravity, as in the Curl-Up itself. Its tone is therefore important in maintaining the normal spinal curves and preventing a hollow back and a great deal of mechanical malfunction. The *oblique* Curl-Ups strengthen primarily the oblique abdominal muscles which form the diagonal bands of the abdominal corset and which wrap round the waist and over the abdomen. In strengthening them you are thus improving your waistline as well as firming your abdomen.

Notes

1 If you can curl down but find it difficult to come up to the sitting position, lower your knees a little, though still keeping your soles flat on the ground. Or use an easier hand position.

2 If you simply cannot manage the Curl-Ups – if you collapse down and cannot make it up at all – practice first curling back and up just a little way, always keeping your back rounded. As you curl back you will discover a 'balancing point', the point of no return beyond which, if your muscles are weak, you lose control and collapse. Curl back just to that point, and up again. With practice you will find the balancing point ever closer to the ground. Once you go beyond the 45° point, half-way, the abdominal muscles are working. Until you are able to reach 45° the curl-back is just a preparatory exercise. (With this partial curl-back you may feel some strain on your legs. Just ignore it.)

3 If even this is difficult, lie on your back, low back dropping to the ground, knees bent. Lift your head to look at your knees and then lower it. If you place your hands on your abdomen you will feel how the muscles there are brought into play. Again, strengthen the three directions, looking up straight to your knees and then to either side. (If you have a stiff neck you may experience quite a strong pull on raising your head. This is nothing to worry about – the action is in fact quite helpful for tight neck muscles.)

23 Low- Back Stretch

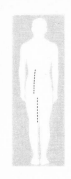

Stretches low back and inside thigh

Sit with your knees bent, soles of the feet together. Place your fingertips on the ground in front of you. With relaxed shoulders . . . creep your fingertips forward. Breathe easily. Creep them further forward. And further.

When the limit is reached, retract your abdomen hard and let your fingertips slide still further forward. Release. (Repeat.)

Pull your feet as close to your body as possible, letting your knees fall outwards. Drop your shoulders, keeping them low and loose. The aim is to 'walk' your fingertips as far forward as you can, thus rounding and stretching your low back. When you have reached your apparent limit, pull your abdomen in really hard and slide

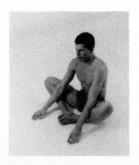
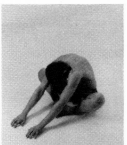

just a bit further forward still. Whenever you contract one group of muscles hard, the opposite group (the antagonists) relax. Here, with the abdominal muscles tight, their antagonists in the low back relax and you gain a few extra degrees of movement.

The Benefit
This helps to stretch and impart flexibility to the low back in the safest possible way. (Touching the toes with straight knees also loosens the back, but is potentially hazardous.) Allowing your knees to fall out to the sides helps stretch tight inner thigh muscles and loosen the hips.

Cautions
1 If this forward bending still produces pain in the low back despite the bent legs, omit the exercise.
2 Omit the movement also if you have an over-flat low back (no concave curve at all when you stand, and no 'bottom').
3 Only tighten your abdominal muscles at the very end of the movement. To hold them in for too long could constrict the organs, raise the blood pressure and interfere with the breathing.

24 Twisting Low-Back Stretch

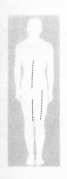

Stretches low back, inside thigh and back of thigh

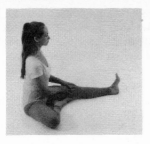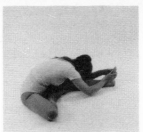

Sit on the ground, back straight, one leg stretched to the side, the other leg bent – sole of foot to opposite thigh. Place your thumbs on top of the straight knee, fingers loosely circling the leg.

Turn your shoulders in line with the straight leg. Keeping your back straight . . . slide your hands a little way towards your foot. Breathe easily. Slide a little further. And a little further. At the limit of the movement, pull in your abdomen and reach a little further forward still. Release and straighten. (Repeat on alternate sides.)

Check that you are sitting on your sitting bones, and not slouching back on your tailbone. Let your back support itself so your ribcage is well up out of your waistline, your back at a right-angle to the floor. Separate your legs so they are as wide apart as you can manage and then bend one leg bringing the foot as close to the body as you can, sole anchored against opposite thigh, knee relaxing out to the side. (If this is easy, you can put your foot on top of the thigh of the straight leg.) Turn your shoulders hard round so your body is in line with the straight leg and you are facing your foot. (If at any point you find the straight leg bending at all, push the heel away and pull the toes towards you.) The aim is now to ease yourself forward – chest to foot, *not* head to knee. Stay well up out of your waistline to maintain the length of your lower body and, keeping your spine straight, slide your hands a little way towards your foot. Breathe easily. Drop your shoulders. The releasing of the shoulders and the letting go of the breath relax the body, helping you to gain more movement more comfortably. Slide a little further forward again. Check that you are still well up out of your waistline. Slide forward a little further still – and further. Finally, pull in your abdomen hard and let yourself stretch forward just a fraction more. The eventual aim is to link your hands around your instep or even further forward in front of your foot, and to lie your body flat along your leg.

The Benefit
The benefits to the back from this stretch are identical to the simple Low-Back Stretch (no.23), but a much stronger stretch is produced on either side. Any inequality in the muscle lengths of the right and left sides will probably be reflected in the ease with which you can do the exercise to each side. If the spinal support muscles are shortened on one side, there is likely to be scoliosis (a sideways spinal curvature), convex to the opposite side. This will mostly be mild, probably undetected, but the body will nevertheless be imbalanced from side to side and suffer a degree of mechanical strain. So if you find you cannot get as close to the one foot as to the other, work hard on the stiff side in order to restore the equilibrium and straighten out your spine. A corresponding stretch on the inside thigh of the bent leg and the back of the thigh of the straight leg also eases tight muscles there, and loosens the hips.

Cautions
1 This movement cannot – and must not – be forced. It may take weeks, months or even years, but gradually the back tension will release and you will be able to perform it easily.
2 Tighten your abdomen only at the very end of the movement in order to avoid any strain.

Note
This exercise may appear to contradict the warning that touching your toes with your legs straight may well cause back trouble, but in fact there is no anomaly. In reaching towards the left foot, for example, the *left* back-thigh muscles and *right* low-back muscles are stretched, and vice versa to the other side. The two sets of muscles on the same side are not, therefore, pulling against each other.

25 Head-and-Shoulder Raise

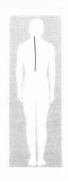

Strengthens upper back

Lie on your front, head resting on your forehead, arms relaxed by your sides. Stretch your feet back as far as you can and, keeping your chin tucked in, lift your head and shoulders. Breathe easily. Lift more.

Now brace back your shoulders. Hold. Lift. Slowly lower. (Repeat.)

Adjust your position so you are in as long a line as possible. 'Lengthen' your legs but keep them relaxed, sinking into the ground. The idea is to lift and strengthen the *upper* back – there should be no strain or pain in the low back. If you feel that the effort is being taken by your low back, 'walk' your feet away from you, elongating your legs still more. This will stretch you out under your hips, giving you firm contact with the ground and a stable base from which to extend the upper back or thorax.

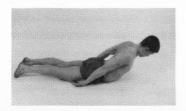

The degree of thoracic backward bend is actually very limited because it is restricted by the shape and contact of the bones. The most you can hope to achieve is about a straight line of the upper spine and there is therefore a tendency to cheat, in two ways. One is to arch the more mobile lower back, even to lift the legs, the other is to arch the neck by throwing back the head. Either of these gives a false feeling of upper-back lift. Keep your legs 'long' and let both arms and legs relax into the ground. Rest your head on your forehead, not your chin, and maintain this length at the back of the neck throughout the lift. This means you will be looking down at the ground, not up, ahead of you. Whilst you will not, cannot, achieve much more than a straight line, the *feeling* is one of an actual back-bend, and you should be able to clear your lower ribs from the ground. This is a strenuous exercise and the breathing is crucial in order not to feel tired. Let your breathing be loose and easy. Allow each outbreath. It is often helpful to lift on the inbreath. Sustain the lift for a few breaths and lift a little further, again on an inbreath. Sustain, allowing the outbreaths, and lift. Sustain and lift once more. At the limit of the lift, brace back your shoulders and hold for a few more breaths.

The Benefit
Whilst there is a normal, very slight, rounding of the upper spine, it *is* only slight. In the standing position the back should appear virtually straight. Often, though, the upper back becomes over-rounded, its convexity compensating for, and being compensated by, excessive concave curves of the low back and neck. The convexity indicates weakness, and the concavity tension and shortening, of the spinal support muscles – the strong cords of muscle that run either side of the spine. The Head-and-Shoulder Raise helps to strengthen the muscles which support the upper area of the spine, holding it gracefully erect. Additionally, there is often a tendency to rounding *across* the back, leading to round shoulders. The bracing of the shoulders helps to counteract this. Both the lift and the brace work very strongly, as the action in each case is to lift the weight of the body against gravity.

Caution
Occasionally, there is a *reduced* upper back curve. The upper back is too straight. In this case, omit the exercise.

26 Back Relaxer

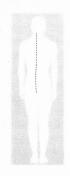

Stretches back

Kneel back on your heels, arms loosely by your sides. Keeping your chin on your chest . . . lean forward to rest your head on the ground. Breathe easily. Relax.

Now stretch your fingertips forward along the ground. And more. Slowly come to the upright position. (Repeat.)

Your bottom should rest on your heels and the top of your head on the ground. If at first you cannot manage to drop your head or heels right down, relax into the position as far as you can, then on an outbreath drop a little further. Stay with it. Breathe yourself down, using the outbreaths to help you. If you find you can drop bottom or head right down but not both together, settle back on to your heels first, then the head – because of its weight – will be eased down more quickly by gravity. Before straightening up,

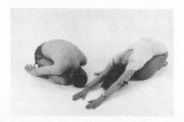

stretch your arms forward into the 'Moslem prayer position'. Creep your fingers as far forward as you can, as this will help to give a good stretch to any tight muscles around your chest and shoulders.

The Benefit
After the strenuous effort of a back bend such as the Head-and-Shoulder Raise (no.24) this forward bend relaxes muscles which have been working hard. Any forward bend would do the same thing, but this way is particularly pleasant once you can do it. You will soon become more supple and, when mastered, you will find this movement enormously soothing and relaxing, perhaps because you are virtually in a foetal position (hence its yoga name, 'pose of the child'). It is also helpful for anyone who has an over-flat upper back with tight contracted muscles. By the time both bottom and head are able to drop right down, the tense upper back will be considerably relaxed.

Caution
Do not force pain in the knees. If it does hurt your knees, lie on your side instead, then curl into a ball. You will gain more or less the same benefit.

27 Waistline Firmer

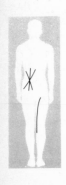

Strengthens back, abdomen and inside thigh

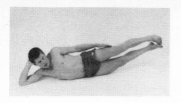

Lie on one side, propping your head with your hand and resting your other arm along the upper side of your body. Lift both legs together, as high as you can. Hold. Breathe easily. Lift more. Slowly lower. (Repeat on alternate sides.)

Make sure you are well on your side, neither rolling forward nor back. Your legs should be in line with your body – which means they should be far enough back for you not to be able to see your toes or your knees. Keep your legs together as you lift. If your hip bone presses painfully into the floor, adjust your position so you are more comfortable. It may be easier at first to place your free hand on the ground in front of you for support. Once you have lifted your legs and gained control of your balance, place the arm along the upper side of your body.

The Benefit
This exercise strengthens the abdominal and back muscles of the upper side and helps to trim the waistline on that side. The inside thigh of the lower leg is also firmed and strengthened. If there is a sideways curvature, however slight, in the low back, concentrate on strengthening the weak side. For example, if there is a spinal curve convex to the left, lie on your right side and lift your legs to the left. This will tighten the weak left side, helping to bring it into balance with the right. Simultaneously, the aim should be to stretch the tight right side. For this you can do the standing Side Bend (no.28), but only to the left.

28 Side Bend

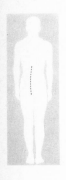

Loosens lower spine, stretches back and sides

Stand with your feet a little way apart, toes pointing forward. Lift your arms sideways and above your head. Link your fingers. Turn your palms up to face the sky, pushing up hard so your arms are straight.

Lean to the side. Lean further. Breathe easily. Lean further still. Straighten. (Repeat on alternate sides.)

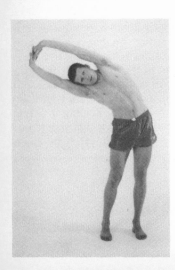

Your feet should stay parallel and not turn out. Let your arms stretch fully but keep your shoulders relaxed and low. Lift up out of your waistline. As you bend, make sure there is no twist of your body, and that you are not cheating by pushing your hip out to the side, leaning forward or turning. This is a pure sideways movement. Allow your head to drop right over. You may feel a really strong stretch down your side. Go with it, using your breathing to help you. Hold the position on each incoming breath. Bend a little more on the outgoing breath.

The Benefit
Side bending from an upright position will help give you a beautifully supple spine, especially in the low back and neck where the movement is not restricted by the ribcage. It will help normalize the length of any tight slips of muscle which may be restricting mobility in the spine. (If you want to use sideways bending to improve your waistline, do the Waistline Firmer, no.27. There you are in effect achieving a side bend by lifting your legs *against* gravity, and the effect is therefore mainly a strengthening and firming one. This exercise, where you go *with* gravity, helps you to be more supple.) Note that if there is any sideways curvature in the low back, the aim should be to stretch one side only until the body is brought into alignment. For example, if there is a spinal curve convex to the left, just do the side bends to the left. This will *stretch* the tight right side. At the same time the Waistline Firmer should be used to *strengthen* the weak left side, by lying on your right and lifting your legs up to the left.

Caution
If you have high blood pressure, heart problems or feel dizzy, keep your arms low. You can, for example, put your hands on your hips. Or you can let them hang loose by your sides. In this case you should be able to bend far enough to touch the outside of your knee with your fingertips, still maintaining a pure sideways bend with no twist.

29 Trunk Rotation

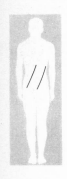

Loosens upper spine, strengthens abdomen

Stand with your feet a little way apart, toes facing forwards. Lift your arms sideways and above your head. Link your fingers. Turn your palms up to face the sky, pushing up hard so your arms are straight. Turn to one side as far as you can. Turn more. Breathe easily. Turn still more. Release. (Repeat on alternate sides.)

Keep your feet parallel and your weight evenly balanced. Your weight, as always, should be taken evenly between the heels and the balls of the feet. Take care not to let your ankle roll in on the side away from which you are turning. Do not resist the movement with your head. Turn, shoulders *and* head, to look right round behind you. As a variation, cross the left foot over the right and with your arms above your head as before, turn to the left. Repeat to the other side.

The Benefit
The twisting aids flexibility of the spine, especially in the thoracic or upper-back area where rotation is most free. It also helps strengthen the oblique abdominal muscles. Crossing the feet helps stabilize the legs and pelvis and isolates the movement to the upper spine. It also provides some resistance to the movement, increasing the strengthening effect for the abdominal and spinal rotation muscles.

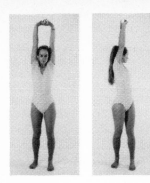 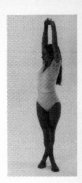

Caution

If you have high blood pressure, heart problems or feel dizzy, keep your arms low. For example, put your hands on your hips, or grip the fingers of the two hands behind your waist. You can help the loosening of your spine by pushing with one hand.

30 The Twist

Loosens spine, stretches — opens up — chest

Lie on your left side, propping your head on your left hand. Bend your right leg (knee to ground, instep to left knee). Grasp your right knee with your left hand (head on the ground, right hand in front of your face).

Now stretch your right arm forward – and up to the vertical – and behind you, following the movement with your head. Breathe easily. Return again to the starting position. (Repeat on alternate sides.)

Make sure you are well on your side, not rolling forward or backward. Your legs should be in line with your body. (Remember that this is usually further back than you think – you should not be able to see your knees or your toes.) Check that your head is also in line. As you bend your upper leg, drop your knee to the ground and anchor the sole of your foot against the other knee. Clasp your bent knee with the hand that was supporting your head and rest your head on the ground, still in line with your body. (The bent knee, held by your hand, remains on the ground throughout the movement, stabilizing the pelvis.) Keep your free arm at shoulder level, palm down, as you stretch it forward slowly and fully, then up in the air and, palm up, back to the ground behind you, describing as large an arc of movement as you can. Really stretch. Follow your hand with your eyes to allow a full spinal twist. If the whole of the arm and shoulder do

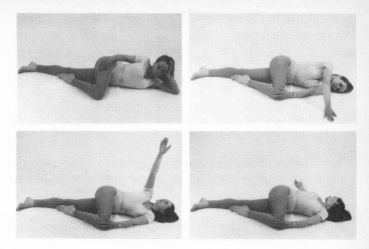

not fall right back to the ground, simply allow them to release a little further with each outbreath. If there is pain in the shoulder, modify by bending your arm. You should eventually be able to hold this position for several minutes, provided you breathe easily and relax into it. Finally, return to the starting position, arm curled on the ground in front of your face. This provides a relaxing countertwist.

The Benefit
This movement relaxes the back, helping to restore suppleness to the spine, and is beneficial to health, appearance and mobility and for the release of tension. It sometimes helps to ease a backache and is always worth a try if your back is hurting. You may hear the click – click – click of your vertebrae as you twist back in what amounts almost to a gentle, and very safe, spinal manipulation. The exercise will also help restore the normal length to shortened chest muscles, which can lead to shallow breathing, round shoulders and restricted arm movement.

31 Knee Push

'First aid' for backache

Lie on your back. Bend one knee to your chest. Clasp your hands loosely over your bent knee.

Keeping your head level . . . push your knee away against your hands. Breathe easily. Push harder. Release. (Repeat with alternate legs.)

Push your knee away as hard as you can against the resistance of your hands, so your arms are pulled straight. Make sure your other leg remains firmly on the ground. (If it wants to bend, push your heel away, pull your toes towards you and brace your knee down flat.) Do not hold your breath. Allow the outbreath. The exercise only achieves its effect if you maintain an unstrained posture of the head. Rest on the base of your skull, face parallel with the ceiling, back of the neck parallel with the floor. Your head may want to roll back, chin in the air, as you push your knee, but if you allow this to happen all the curves of the spine are affected and the movement loses its value.

The Benefit
This first aid measure for pain in the low back is not absolutely guaranteed to help but very often it will relieve the spasm which *is* the backache and it can be wonderfully soothing. It is always worth a try if your back hurts or feels tired.

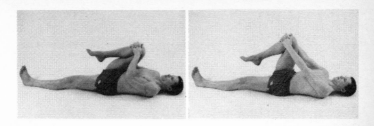

Caution
Avoid the exercise if it actually *provokes* pain in the low back.

HEADLINES

(Head and neck)

The head is heavy, about 12 pounds in weight. The neck muscles, accustomed to constantly supporting it, are consequently rarely weak. On the contrary, they frequently overwork. They are tense. Nowhere in the body do we store tension more than in the neck and shoulders. The habitually tense muscles shorten and thicken, restricting head movement and sometimes causing headaches. In the human being it is common for the head/neck relationship to be permanently out of kilter. As a result of the human upright position the head is in delicate balance anyway, supported by the muscles and ligaments to which it is attached. If these muscles are working too hard – as, unfortunately, they often are – they pull the head out of alignment. For most people, therefore, the purpose of neck exercises is to *stretch* and relax tight muscles.

The beneficial effect of stretching short, tense neck muscles is far-reaching, for if the head sits awkwardly on the shoulders the entire postural 'set' of the body will be affected. F. M. Alexander viewed the head/neck relationship as being the primary control for the coordination of the body. When this relationship is disturbed – when the head is out of alignment – general body functioning, indeed the whole psychophysical balance, is impaired. A falling cat usually lands safely on its feet. First its head-righting reflexes right the head, then a reflex chain-reaction corrects the rest of the body. Where the head leads, the body follows.

Investigations of the 'startle pattern' (the response to an unexpected or alarming stimulus) show first a distortion of the head/neck/torso relationship – head forward, neck shortened and arched backwards. Then, if the stimulus is strong enough, there is a hunching of the shoulders, followed by a flattening of the chest and finally by a bending of the knees. The whole sequence from neck to knees, if carried right through, takes about half a second. What is interesting is that anxiety, pain, fear, depression and

The Ideal

Common Deviations

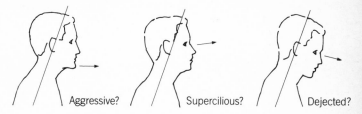

Aggressive?   Supercilious?   Dejected?

32, **33** (see also introductory section on Posture)

fatigue all reproduce virtually the same postural deviations. But, unlike the sudden startle response and its immediate release once the stimulus has passed, the pattern of tension in a nervous or dejected person is sustained over long periods – can, indeed, remain as a permanent postural aberration. Muscles adapt and shorten, so 'fixing' the poor alignment. In our stressful culture the whole pattern of shortening is so frequent in the elderly as to be generally accepted – wrongly – as an intrinsic feature of aging.

Whatever survival value the startle pattern may have as a response to an emergency, as a continuing reaction to negative feelings it appears to be wholly maladaptive, depriving the structure of its flexibility, interfering with breathing, affecting the eyesight. The tension involved in contracting the back of the neck into a shortened position actually maintains, even creates, psychological tension. If you observe, you will see how, for many people, every new movement – standing up from a chair, stepping off a kerb, changing direction – is initiated by a jerking back of the head. It is as though the chin has to lift in order to heave the body into the new position. Ideally, movement should proceed from the 'centre', and it is always graceful and coordinated when it does. The neck then remains free and undisturbed and the head (and the person) well balanced.

Norms of Movement

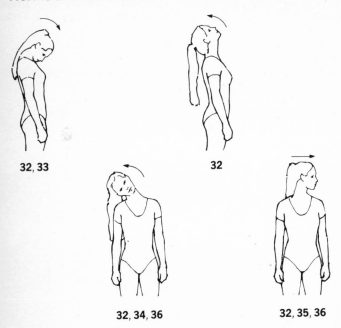

32, 33　　　　　　**32**

32, 34, 36　　　　　**32, 35, 36**

The head/neck relationship is not static but dynamic. We are not rigid statues. One can lift one's face, for example, to look at the stars without any disruption of harmony. It is the constant, unconscious throwing back of the head – the arched neck, the jutting chin, the upturned face – which betokens disharmony and gives an, often false, impression of arrogance or hostility.

Before all else, practising the Head Balance (no.32) will help rectify the pattern of shortening. It can be used any time, anywhere, for freeing the neck. All the neck exercises (and in fact *all* the sitting and standing exercises) will be performed more beneficially and with less effort if preceded by the Head Balance – just as the lying exercises will be performed more effectively if the head rests on the *base* of the skull with the neck long and flat at the back. The Head Balance, however, is not just a preparation for exercises. It is a point of focus which, together with the grounding and centring, can be returned to again and again during the day.

The other exercises in this section all require very slow, very smooth movement. The neck, though immensely strong, has a delicate framework of small intricate bones and many tiny slips of muscle. It needs respect and gentleness. Quick jerky movements are ineffectual as exercise – they will never increase the range of movement of your neck and they can make you dizzy. Done slowly, these movements relax and invigorate you. They can be practised in any position, but perhaps the best way is sitting on the floor. In every case only your *head* moves. Your shoulders stay still, your body motionless. Their purpose is to free your neck so that head movements can be smooth and graceful.

32 Head Balance

Starting point for all sitting and standing exercises

Sit or stand well up out of your waistline, back straight, head level. Lift your shoulders a very little. Roll them back. Press them down. Keeping them down, release the pressure. Breathe easily. Maintain.

You are aiming to allow the neck to achieve its full normal length, which will give you a lovely feeling of poise and balance. First find the ideal set of your shoulders which, if really relaxed, automatically assume a backward, downward posture. Lift them a fraction first. Roll them back. Press them down, then release so that they remain low but at ease. You will feel a contrasting pull at the back of the neck. Check in the mirror, and if one shoulder is higher than the other work a little extra on the high shoulder.

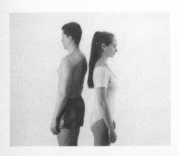
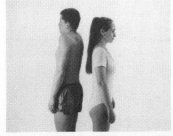

Direct the back of your neck *back* until your earlobes are in line with the point of your shoulders, your nose in line with your navel. Then feel yourself as if suspended, like a puppet whose string is attached to the back of its head. With this stretch, the spine of your neck will straighten and lengthen, ironing out any visible hollowing behind the neck. Your chin will adopt its ideal neutral position, neither poking up nor pulling tightly in. Your breastbone will lift. Your eye level will drop to the correct position. (Do not, however, arch your lower back.) The object is graceful relaxation, not stiff military rigidity. So if with all this upward stretching you feel literally up-tight, 'stuck' in your chest, drop your awareness to your body's centre of gravity, a couple of inches below your navel, and 'centre' yourself there. Feel the calmness. Be aware of the rise and fall of your abdomen as you breathe. Let yourself be grounded, too. If you are standing, *feel* the ground with your feet.

A beautifully poised head is perhaps best typified by a tribesgirl carrying a water jug on her head. The back of her neck is long and straight, her earlobes well back in line with her shoulders, her chin level, her breastbone high. She looks directly ahead, not up in the air. As head balance is of prime importance in the alignment and coordination of the body as a whole, she seems to glide smoothly, loosely, easily. Try it. Put a book on your head. Walk. Change directions. As soon as your head loses its perfect balance, the book will fall off. The aim is to rediscover this same natural elegance – it is your birthright too.

The Benefit
The Head Balance helps overcome problems caused by malalignment of the head and adaptive shortening of the neck muscles. It will give you a longer and more graceful neck, prevent or

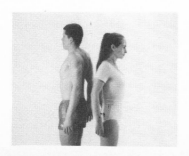
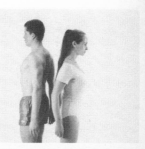

improve a double chin and, in overcoming stiffness, tension and resultant thickening of the neck muscles, lessen tension headaches and neck and shoulder pain. The whole body will be more coordinated, and your very sense of your body will be heightened. In women, the breasts will be shapelier and firmer, and in men the physique of the upper torso will correspondingly improve. Breathing will deepen, and the voice will increase in resonance (neck tension can be responsible for a weak or hoarse voice). Even vision may improve, since when the head is thrown back and the eye level raised, the eyes become strained. The Head Balance is not so much an exercise as a way of finding the optimum alignment of the head. With the head nicely poised you will be fitter, look better and have a wonderful sensation of tranquillity, lightness and freedom.

Note

As a headache reliever, exaggerate the rolling up, back and down
of your shoulders, then – keeping
your head and neck in line – link
your hands behind your back and
push them down as far as you can.
This often works like magic.

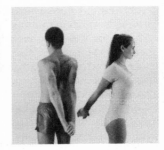

33 Neck Relaxer

Stretches back of neck

Sit or stand well up out of your waistline, back straight, head level. Drop your chin to your chest. Interlace your fingers and place them on top of your head. Let your elbows hang down loosely. Rest in that position. Breathe easily.

Remove your hands. Slowly uncurl until your head is level. (Repeat.)

Sit upright with your shoulders low, slightly back, and relaxed. Do not let your back collapse when you drop your head forward. Your chin should touch your chest, so that the muscles at the back of the neck are stretched and therefore (although it may not feel like it) relaxed. With each exhalation allow the head – and

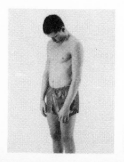
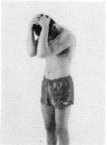

the shoulders – to drop a little further, but keep your back straight. Check your elbows. They should fall *down*, simply hanging by their own weight, and not stick out to the sides or forwards. Adjust your hand position so you feel the maximum stretch. Relax there, aware of the stretch, observing the rhythm of your breathing. Maintain the stretch as you take your hands away, feeling the weight of your head as it hangs down. Then, very very slowly, uncurl your neck, vertebra by vertebra, from the base of the neck upwards until your head is effortlessly balanced.

The Benefit

With your hands you are merely applying a passive stretch, a little gentle overpressure to the muscles behind the neck. These are the muscles that arch the neck and head backwards, thus lifting the chin and raising the eye level. They are often chronically tense and short, always working, never relaxed. The sustained stretch helps lengthen and relax them and is marvellously soothing.

Caution

Dropping the head forward *and* tilting it back is often practised as an exercise. If you do this, take great care with the backward movement. Never force it or do it sharply. It is the whiplash position. And never tilt your head back without opening your mouth, or the delicate tissues in front of the throat will be stretched and slackened, predisposing towards a double chin.

34 Head Sideways Tilt

Stretches side of neck

Sit or stand well up out of your waistline, back straight, head level. Tilt your head sideways, ear to shoulder. Breathe easily. Tilt more. And more. Straighten. (Repeat on alternate sides.)

This is a pure sideways tilt of the head. Tilt but do *not* turn. Only your head moves, always facing forward, chin not poking up or down. (To avoid turning, keep your eyes on one spot, straight ahead.) Your body should remain still and upright, with no sideways bend at the waist. Your shoulders stay level and down. Do not lift your shoulder up to meet your ear – the movement is 'ear to shoulder', not 'shoulder to ear'. Even more important, the *opposite* shoulder should stay low (in fact, *press* it down, so you

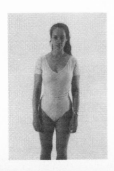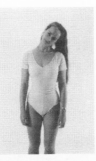

feel the opposing pulls of shoulder and neck). Aim to gain maximum distance from ear to shoulder on the side of the neck away from the tilt. Use your breathing to help you, dropping a little further on the outbreath. Sustain for a few breaths and, keeping your shoulders down, drop again as you exhale. Allow yourself to experience the feeling of stretch which comes if there is any restriction in the side of your neck. It will probably hurt, but it is a good hurt.

The Benefit
Very often there is muscle tension in the neck which restricts head movement. If the side of your neck feels hard and unyielding, or if it is tender to the touch, the side neck muscles are almost certainly tense and probably shortened and thickened. By working at the limit of your present range of movement and putting the muscles on a slow sustained stretch you are actually relaxing the neck (although it may not seem so) and releasing a good deal of tension. As a bonus, your circulation will be opened up, your complexion will glow and you will feel more awake and alive. Tilting to both sides in this way also helps impart flexibility to the spine of the neck. If you are in the habit of holding your head to one side – you may have to check this with a friend, because you will unconsciously straighten when you look in the mirror – then you should do this movement to one side only, to help counteract the shortening which will have occurred. If, for example, you hold your head to the right, the muscles on the right side will be shortened so, to relax them, tilt to the left.

Caution
A strong pull on the outside of your neck (on the side *away* from the tilt) indicates tight muscles which need to be stretched. Do not, however, force pain on the inside (*towards* the tilt) as you may be hurting rather than helping.

35 Head Sideways Turn

Stretches sides and back of neck

Sit or stand well up out of your waistline, back straight, head level. Turn your head slowly to one side. Breathe easily. Turn more. And more. Straighten. (Repeat on alternate sides.)

Let your head swivel very slowly and smoothly to one side, making sure you do not tilt your head or turn your shoulders. Turn but do *not* tilt. Keep your eyes at eye level. (If you find yourself looking at floor or ceiling, then your head is tilted – and remember, eye level itself is often lower after correcting the balance of the head.) Your shoulders should remain facing straight forwards, quite still and, as always, relaxed and low. Stay with the limit of the movement. Breathe easily. On an outbreath

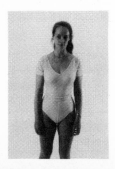
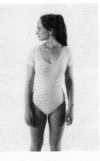

turn a little further. Sustain for a few breaths and turn still more. By staying with it and using the exhalation for your turn, you can push back your limits, limits which generally speaking are nothing more than tight tense muscles. Full movement is a 90° turn, shoulders and body square to the front, a perfect profile to the side. When you have turned as far as possible, release and let the head straighten, more or less of its own accord.

The Benefit
Turning to one side, aiming to push back the barriers to mobility, helps relax the muscles whose job it is to turn the head to the other side. The whole side-to-side movement, done slowly, helps the flexibility of the neck. If, for example, you are a car driver, free side-to-side movement is essential for speed of reaction and safety.

36 Head Tilt and Turn

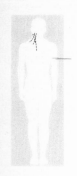

Stretches sides and back of neck

Sit or stand well up out of your waistline, back straight, head level. Drop your shoulders. Tilt your head to the right, ear to shoulder. Breathe easily. Tilt more.

Then, maintaining the tilt . . . turn very slowly to look up to the left. Then down to the right. And up – slowly – and down. Straighten your head to the vertical. (Repeat to the other side.)

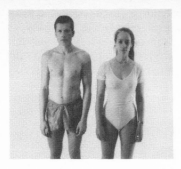 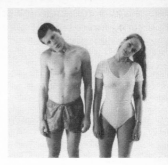

Keeping your body straight, your face forwards and your shoulders down, do the Head Sideways Tilt (no.34) to the right. Very slowly indeed, maintaining the tilt, turn your head to look as far up to the left as you can – and a little bit further. Then, describing as large an arc of movement as possible, turn to look down to the right – and further – always using your breathing to help you. Repeat slowly several times, diagonally up and down. Straighten your head. Tilt to the left and repeat. This is not a circling or a rolling of the head. The head does not drop back.

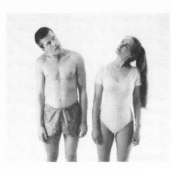 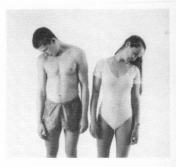

Rather, it is a semi-circle, a half-moon movement. The chin sweeps the chest as you look up to the sky and it sweeps the chest again as you look down at the ground. If there is tension in the neck, you will feel all manner of pulls and stretches. Allow – 'go into' – every little stretch.

The Benefit
The slow, slow execution of this tilt-and-turn helps stretch and

relax the numerous large and small muscles in the neck – all lying at slightly different angles, acting in slightly different ways – where tension is often stored, even generated. It avoids the grinding of the bones and the dizziness sometimes associated with the more usual head circling, but provides a much more powerful release for the muscles.

FACE FACTS

(The face)

In 1927, Elinor Glyn, a novelist, a beauty and a legend in her own time, published *The Wrinkle Book*. It is an evocatively written manual of facial exercises and as such has probably never been bettered. Given the date it was written it is a remarkable little volume, applying to the face principles that are in accordance with the most up-to-date muscle-shaping techniques. Usually, however, the type of resisted exercises she advocates have been used only to firm up the body, while faces are allowed to drop and droop as they will.

Observing that the aging face tends to 'droop forwards and downwards towards the central points of the nose, mouth and chin', Elinor Glyn developed a whole range of exercises to counteract these tendencies. Perhaps the most interesting among them is a set of exercises she calls the 'Auricular Series', so named because they depend on the ability to wiggle the ears. Without realizing it, she had stumbled on an age-old yogic method of facial rejuvenation. Moving the ears is, for most of us, a lost capacity, but the mechanism is still there and can be brought under voluntary control surprisingly easily. With a little practice is becomes possible to move the ears both upwards and backwards. The ears draw the tissues of the face up and back with them, improving muscle tone and smoothing away wrinkles by producing the effect of a face lift *from within*.

The most basic 'face lift' technique is not an exercise at all, but simply a way of relaxing the forehead. It does not involve control of the ears, but forms an integral part of the other techniques which do, and it can be done whenever you think of it, wherever you are. For this, with eyes and mouth very soft and tongue relaxed, imagine your eyes are wide apart – so wide-set that they are at the side of your face, even beyond your face. Do not *do* anything. Just visualize. There is no limit to how far apart your eyes can be in your imagination. The mere act of imagining in this way will relax tension in your forehead and miraculously iron out any vertical scowl lines between your eyebrows. At the same time, allowing a softness in the mouth and eyes will immediately make you feel gentler, kinder and more sensitive to other people.

The two techniques which follow and which are, like the one described here, ancient yogic practices, are ear-wiggling exercises similar to those recommended by Elinor Glyn. The first one helps counteract the horizontal forehead lines and lift the facial contours upwards. The other acts on the vertical nose-mouth-chin folds. It smoothes and lifts the face outwards, away from the centre. Visualization of the smooth firm face you desire forms an intrinsic part of these methods.

37 Face Lift (Up)

Strengthens muscles of face

Imagine your eyes very wide apart. Raise your ears, and simultaneously . . . draw your forehead up and your scalp back. Breathe easily. Up more . . . back more. Release. (Repeat.)

To begin with, it is best to practise this lift in front of a mirror. Keep your face quiet and serene and free of tension. You are aiming to train muscles which are often not immediately under voluntary control. All the other facial muscles – the ones you use all the time and can move at will – should remain quite relaxed. Visualizing wide-set eyes will aid this general facial relaxation. Now, with a tranquil face, raise your ears. Probably, nothing at all will happen the first time, or the second, or the third. It helps

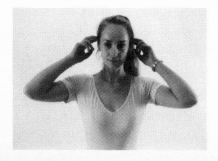

therefore to put your fingers on top of your ears. You can then *feel* the smallest response, the tiniest twitch of movement. At first this may be only a flicker, later quite a visible lift.

The forehead and scalp are covered by one continuous sheet of muscle from the eyebrows to the hairline at the back of the head. As you raise your ears, aim to draw this muscle sheet up over your forehead, smoothing out any horizontal furrows, and back over the top of your head right down to the base of the skull. Again, nothing will appear to happen at first. Later, with practice, the lift should be such that the tissues of the whole face are slightly raised – you should even feel the pull under your chin. Do not tire the muscles. Just do it once or twice, holding each contraction for only a couple of seconds. As the muscles become used to working again, you can perform the lift more frequently. Eventually you can actually resist the ear movement with your fingers so the muscles work harder and strengthen more.

The Benefit
This exercise will help keep your face young and firm. If you start before any sagging has occurred you will not, of course, actually notice any difference, but if you feel a need to improve your facial contours and the smoothness of your skin the exercise can help a great deal. Not only will it tend to smooth out any horizontal forehead frown lines, it will lift the whole face from within. Initially there will be little noticeable change. Later there will probably be an appreciable effect during the contraction. Eventually, as muscle tone improves, the results will become increasingly marked and long-lasting. Be patient. Do not expect miracles overnight. If you persevere, ultimate results promise to be finer than any surgical facelift.

38 Face Lift (Out)

Strengthens muscles of face

Imagine your eyes very wide apart. Move your ears back, and simultaneously . . . draw back your scalp and the tissues of your face. Breathe easily. Pull back more . . . and more . . . towards the centre-back of your skull. (Repeat.)

First, help release all the tension in your facial expression muscles by visualizing wide-set eyes. (As for the previous exercise, use a mirror in the early stages.) With your face quite calm, direct your ears backwards towards the back of your head. *Feel* them, or at first *imagine* them, moving backwards. If, as is likely, nothing seems to happen the first few times, persevere. Place your fingertips on your ears so you can detect the slightest response.

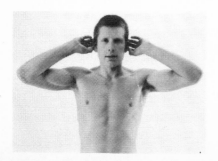

Surprisingly soon you will sense the first flicker of movement, and once that happens you have something to work on. As you draw back your ears, feel as if you are also retracting the scalp towards the middle of the back of your head. Then, when you start to gain mastery over your scalp and ears, visualize the tissues of your face also being drawn back with your ears, out and away from your nose, mouth and chin. Do not overdo it – little and often is the better way. Tiring the muscles may hinder rather than assist progress. When finally it becomes easier to draw back the scalp, ears and facial muscles, use your fingers to resist the movement. The muscles will work harder and the effect will be enhanced.

The Benefit
Tiny and at first imperceptible as this movement is, it will help counteract the inward sag of the face, thus smoothing out the vertical lines – the potentially deep folds that can form from nose to mouth to chin. The face is lifted, out and away from the centre, so that the contours become tauter and firmer.

SHOULDER SHAPERS

(Arm and shoulder)

The lengths of the muscles in the shoulders are every bit as significant as those in the neck in determining the impression of ourselves we unconsciously convey to others – openness or defensiveness, confidence or anxiety, ease with the world or timidity. This is not the body language of gesture, about which so much is written and of which we can become aware, and can to some extent control. It is the very structure of our body which is speaking for us.

To a large degree we create our bodies for ourselves. Obviously, there are givens. No conscious procedure or unconscious mechanism is going to significantly change our height, the length of our limbs, or a million and one other individual characteristics. But the set of the shoulders, the shape of the chest, the figure, is a personal imprint of our own moulding. Often it is, in fact, not so much that we build our body as that we inhibit its own natural harmonious development. We live in a peculiarly stressful society and we encounter pressure – to be what we are not, to conform, to attain – at a very tender age. We may be so suppressed in infancy that we come to expect

The Ideal

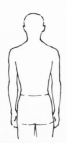

Common Deviations

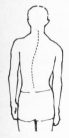

One shoulder low
Spinal curvature
Pelvis high
17

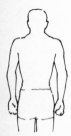

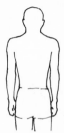

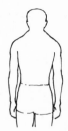

Shoulders high
(overdeveloped athletic type)

Shoulders high
(anxious type)

Round shoulders

12 (arms above head), **20** (arms above head), **25**, **26** (arms in front), **30**, **32**, **33**, **34**, **35**, **36**, **40**, **41**, **42**

restriction for the rest of our lives. No wonder that we cannot cope easily, that we lift our shoulders to protect ourselves, or hold our breath in order not to feel. Unfortunately, these maladaptive responses become, in time, a way of life. The muscles which produce them work too hard too often. The wrong muscles undergo a rigorous body-building programme of their own, out of balance with the rest of the body. They change their length and tone. They shorten and thicken and become hard. They become a cage, making appropriate response to fresh stimuli, and subsequent release, impossible. We are then emotionally as well as physically rigid.

This pattern is only too common, though there are still people who escape it entirely or develop other ways of coping with stress. Use the exercises in this section as tests. If they are effortless for you, and if your shoulders are naturally relaxed and low, you have no problem and there will be something very right and pleasing about your upper body, indeed about you. However, if you discover your movement is restricted and your shoulders are high and hard and lumpy and will not release, you are one of the majority. These shoulder exercises, together with the Head Balance (no.32), will help restore mobility to the shoulder joints, give you more graceful arms, and improve the shape of the chest and breasts, as well as your breathing (and, consequently, general health and state of mind).

Norms of Movement

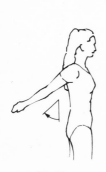

30, 41

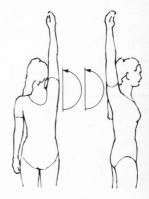

12, 21, 30, 40, 41

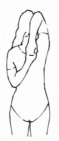

12, 21, 30, 42

You should never forget, though, that it is daily life that matters more than anything else. Always remember, especially when reaching out with your arms, to 'let go' of your shoulders, to let them drop and be loose. (To help relax your shoulders, imagine yourself wearing heavy gloves.) Look in the mirror. If one shoulder is higher than the other, be especially attentive towards that one. Not only will you begin to acquire a much nicer line, you will also help to prevent tension from building up.

39 Arms Backward Lift

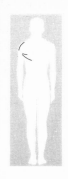

Strengthens shoulder, arm and back

Kneel back on your heels, body and head straight and in line – or stand if this is painful. Interlace your fingers behind your waist. Stretch your arms out behind you. Lift your hands as high as you can. Breathe easily. Stretch and lift. And more.

Now, keeping your hands high . . . drop your chin to your chest and curl your body forward. Breathe easily. Curl further forward. And further still.

Still keeping your hands high . . . slowly uncurl again. Release and lower your arms. (Repeat.)

Be careful not to lean forward, or arch your back, or poke your chin as you stretch your arms behind you. Keep your arms straight and 'long' as you lift them. Enjoy the feeling that your

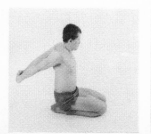

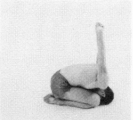

hands are floating up and up, higher and higher. Aim to raise your arms to a right-angle from your body (arms horizontal in the upright position, vertical in the forward curl). Anything less than 50° of lift is restricted. Do not hold your breath – like all movement, it is easier and more pleasurable when you allow the outward breath. When you have lifted your arms fully, bring your elbows as close together as you can. As you curl forward, keep your chin on your chest until the top of your head touches the ground. If you cannot curl over sufficiently – bottom to heels, head to ground – use the outbreath to help you, dropping a little more each time. Once your head does touch the ground, bring it as close to your knees as you can. As you uncurl again, keep your chin on your chest until the last moment. Unroll your spine, vertebra by vertebra, from the tailbone up to the top of your neck.

The Benefit
This exercise strengthens the large back muscle which provides power for the forceful arm movements used in swimming, rowing, chopping wood and the like, and for the vigorous exhalation of singing and laughing. It also helps overcome any stiffness which may make it difficult to put the hands behind the back.

Cautions
1 In curling forward from a standing position, protect your back by relaxing your knees, letting them be loose and slightly bent.
2 Avoid the forward curl in the standing position altogether if you have any back problems.
3 Omit the kneeling position if it forces any pain in the knee-joint. (You can, however, disregard pain on *top* of the thigh, as this merely indicates that the front thigh muscles are too tight – the kneeling will in itself provide a beneficial stretch.)

40 Arms Forward and Above Head

Loosens arm and shoulder

Lie on your back, hands by your sides. Stretch your arms, fingertips to toes. Lift your arms to the vertical, stretching your fingertips upwards. Take them back above your head. Let them fall towards the ground. Let them drop more. And more.

Breathe easily, arms stretched out behind you and in to your ears. On the inbreath – stretch back. On the outbreath – drop down and pull in. Back – down – in. And stretch more. Release. (Repeat.)

The aim is for the arms to come to rest easily on the ground above the head (180° from their 'down' position by the sides), quite straight, upper arms against the ears, elbows relaxing into the ground. The stretch, as you push your fingertips towards your toes before lifting them vertically into the air, separates the bones of the shoulder joint and will allow you to gain more movement than you would without it. Still stretching, take your arms back over your head and for a moment or two just allow them to fall back by their own weight. Make sure that your low back is flat on the ground, or as well down as possible. (If your knees bend, push your heels away and pull your toes towards you.) The position of the head is intimately related to that of the back. Rest on the base, not the top, of the skull, face parallel with the ceiling, back of the neck parallel with the floor, making sure your

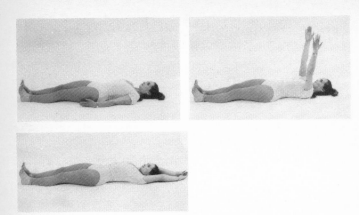

head does not roll back so your chin sticks up in the air. Breathe easily, allowing the outbreath.

If you had time simply to lie there with your arms above your head, the tension would gradually dissolve and your arms would fall back slowly towards the ground. However, to speed the process along, think of the exercise as a two-way stretch and use your breathing to help you. On each inbreath, stretch back, fingertips reaching as far behind you as possible, so your arms lengthen and straighten. Maintaining the stretch, on the outbreath, pull your arms close in to your ears and lower them towards the ground. (Sometimes at this point it is easier to clasp your hands so one arm can help the other.) The important thing is to keep your low back on the ground even if for the moment you appear to gain less movement with your arms. No real increase of flexibility will be achieved if it is at the expense of arching your back. Whether this exercise is exhilarating or exhausting depends on your breathing. If you hold your breath you may feel very tired. If you let go, allowing yourself to breathe out, you will feel wonderfully refreshed.

The Benefit

As well as specifically improving the mobility and gracefulness of the arms and releasing tension stored in the neck and shoulders, this is also a supreme all-over body stretch. For anyone who finds the slightest difficulty in performing it, it is one of the key exercises in the book. All the tight areas at the back are stretched – the backs of the legs, the low back, the neck. The pushing down of the back helps to tone up the abdominal muscles and to straighten out the spine. The ribcage is lifted and the waistline thereby lengthened and neatened. The poise of the head improves, as shortened muscles are eased out to their optimum length. If you enjoy swimming, this arm stretch is an invaluable preparation for the back crawl.

Note
If your arms reach easily back to the ground but your back arches, just work on pressing your back down, keeping your knees straight and head level. The movement then becomes an advanced version of the Pelvic Tilt (no.21).

41 Arms Out and Above Head

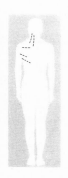

Loosens arm and shoulder

Lie on your back, arms out to the side and resting on the ground, hands at shoulder level, palms up. Stretch your arms outwards. Then, keeping your arms straight . . . slide them flat along the ground towards your ears. And closer. And closer still. Breathe easily. Hold. Release, sliding your hands back to shoulder level. (Repeat.)

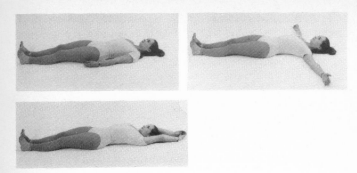

The aim, arms above head (180° from their 'down' position by the sides), is the same as in the previous exercise. Your arms should slide easily along the ground, coming to rest above your head, quite straight, upper arms against your ears, without the elbows rising from the ground or the back pulling into a hollow. Again, lying on your back, drop the small of the back to the ground or as well down as you can. Keep your legs straight and check that your head is resting on the base of the skull, not rolling back so that your neck arches and your chin pokes. Make sure you are not holding your breath. Now, with your hands out to the sides at shoulder level, stretch your fingertips away from you, making your arms as 'long' as possible (so separating the bones of the shoulder joints and allowing greater freedom of movement). Maintain the length in your arms as you slide them a little way towards your ears to a point that is comfortable, and rest there a moment. Check what is happening to your elbows, your knees, your head, your back and your breathing. Slide your arms a little closer to your ears. Pause again. Slide closer still – and closer. When you are as close as you think is possible, alternately work first one arm then the other towards your ear. This way you will gain a few extra degrees of movement. Finally, release to the horizontal and rest for a few seconds.

The Benefit
This exercise stretches muscles which extend from the back and chest to the upper arm. When shortened, as they often are, these muscles tend to hold the arm in to the side so that arm movement is stiff and awkward. Release the muscles and the arms can become fluid and gentle once more. Simultaneously, breathing

deepens and the shape of the upper body improves. The shoulder is a comparatively unstable joint, prone to dislocation and 'frozen shoulder'. Like the others in this section, this exercise helps make it much less vulnerable to injury and strain.

Note
If you are fortunate enough to have free arm movement but your back hollows, slide your arms into the above-head position then work from there to press your back into the ground, using the movement as a back-flattening exercise. You will also be helping to strengthen your abdominal muscles (see Pelvic Tilt, no.21).

42 Hands Clasped Behind Shoulder Blades

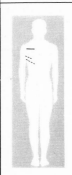

Loosens arm and shoulder

Kneel back on your heels or stand. Place your right hand over your right shoulder (elbow pointing up). Place your left hand behind your waist. Clasp the fingers of the two hands. Pull tight. And tighter still. Breathe easily. Hold. Release. (Repeat on alternate sides.)

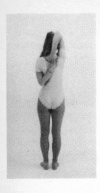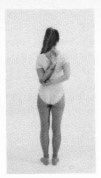

Keep your body straight and your head level. Do not hollow your back or lift your chin. With one hand over your shoulder, the other behind your waist, clasp your hands, pulling the fingers of the two hands tight together. If your fingers do not meet, release the upper hand, put it behind your waist and use it to help lift the lower hand. It is often possible to get the bottom hand much higher up your back by giving it a gentle push. Then *stretch* the upper arm vertically upwards. This will allow the hand to drop further down the back as you reach over the shoulder again. Breathing easily, keep on creeping the fingers along the back towards each other. If they still do not touch, knot a silk scarf three or four times. Take an end in either hand and work from knot to knot, bringing the hands closer and closer. You may find one side much easier than the other. Practise more on the difficult side.

The Benefit
This exercise, like the other arm and shoulder exercises, frees the arms, allowing them to become more graceful and at the same time protecting the shoulder against trauma. It enables the hands to reach behind the back more easily. Tight chest muscles are relaxed, promoting the release of stale air from the lungs and so helping to leave you refreshed and tranquil.

WOMEN ONLY

(Pelvic floor and breasts)

The Pelvic Floor

The pelvic floor is the flat horizontal sheet of muscle between the legs which provides the base support for the pelvic organs – the bladder, the bowel and, in women, the uterus. In fact, 'floor' is not really an entirely apt term – rather, it is a muscular hammock attached to and suspended between two bones, the tailbone at the back and the pubic bone in front, with minor attachments at the sides to the sitting bones. This 'hammock' is pierced vertically by the anus at the back, the urethra (urine canal) in front and centrally by the vagina, which passes down close behind the urethra. It forms a figure-of-eight – one loop (or 'sphincter') slung around the anus, the other around both urethra and vagina – and provides the muscular control for these passages, relaxing during elimination and returning immediately to its normal tone.

To function adequately the pelvic musculature must be firm and flat. Its structure has to be able to withstand the many increases of pressure within the pelvic and abdominal cavities – the intermittent increases produced by laughing, crying, coughing, sneezing, elimination, lifting and so on, and the sustained ever-increasing pressure of pregnancy. The upright stature of the human being has led to a rather flimsy structure compared with that found in animals. The frequent sudden, or not so sudden, increases in pressure from above combined with the pull of gravity from below – intensified because of the human vertical position – encourages the pelvic floor muscles to elongate and sag. They can become weak, too, simply from underuse. Overall fitness has no bearing on their condition, and neither the ordinary activities of daily life nor sports and general exercises provide specific work for them.

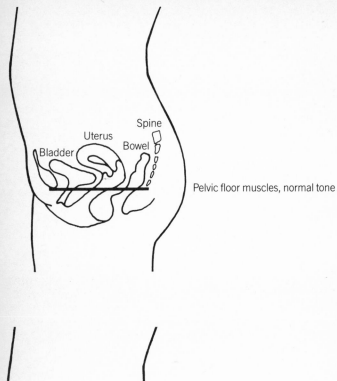

Pelvic floor muscles, normal tone

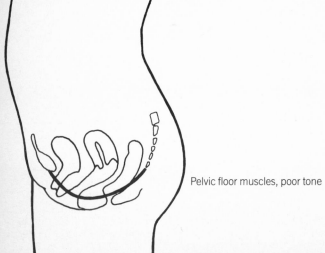

Pelvic floor muscles, poor tone

In women, this proneness of the pelvic floor to sag is aggravated by the innate structural weakness caused by the presence of the vagina, which means that the pelvic floor is pierced by three, rather than two, passages. The front or 'master' sphincter is especially apt to become lax, since it contains both urethra and vagina. If the muscles do sag and drop, the organs they support are displaced, with effects ranging from a sensation simply of fatigue to great discomfort. There may be urinary incontinence, perhaps just a mild dribbling of urine when coughing or sneezing, or real difficulty in control. When the front sphincter is very flabby, it may not be easy to retain a tampon. And long before any of these problems occur, sex may have been ruined for one or both partners because the vagina is insufficiently firm to grip the penis. Needless to say, pregnancy and childbirth, if not counteracted by specific internal exercise, can exacerbate the problem.

However, for all but the most severe cases, the remedy is at hand. The simple set of internal exercises – or pelvic floor contractions – in this section revive a centuries'-old erotic art, the 'sexercises' of the *Arabian Nights* and the *Kama Sutra*, where the ability to grip and release the penis was regarded as a highly prized asset. Still today, certain African tribes do not allow their young girls to marry until they have perfected this control. So the pelvic floor contractions can be done purely as a therapeutic exercise or – even better – they can be done *Kama Sutra* style, when making love.

The Breast

The perennial question fired at exercise teachers is a pleading, 'Have you anything for the bustline?' Whether they feel flat or top heavy, few people seem satisfied with the way they are. Breasts loom large – or miserably small – in our self-image. But while most of us are never likely to match up to the ubiquitous advertisements directed at male fantasies, it is still possible to work towards a more pleasing and satisfying contour.

The breasts are composed of glandular, fibrous and adipose (fatty) tissue. They contain no muscle. Since exercise works on muscle it cannot affect the breasts directly, but the large pectoral muscle is involved directly in determining their shape, position and firmness, and exercise can thus be of considerable help. The Uplift (no.45) given here is *the* classic exercise specifically for the breasts. The shoulder exercises will also help lift and firm you, as well as expanding the chest so that breathing, which is vital, can deepen spontaneously. Another way to help open up the chest wall and restore normal length to tight muscles it to lie relaxed on your back with your hands linked behind your neck and allow your elbows to drop to the floor. If you have difficulty, gently ease them down on each outbreath. If, on the other hand, the movement is easy, you can place a small pillow under your shoulders so that your elbows have further to drop.

Posture, needless to say, is all-important – a notable uplift in front rarely accompanies round shoulders behind. The Head Balance (no.32) can again help in opening out the chest wall so that the breasts can assume their optimum position. And swimming, too, is excellent, because the chest muscles have to work hard against the resistance of the water.

43 Pelvic- Floor Strengthening Exercises

Lie comfortably on your back. Tighten and 'pull up' very slowly the muscles of the anus. Squeeze . . . lift . . . as much as possible. Hold. Breathe easily. Release, slowly and fully.

Contract similarly the muscles of the vagina. Breathe easily. Release.

Tighten the anus and vagina together. Hold. Breathe easily. Pull up more, giving special emphasis to the vagina. Release.

(Repeat.)

To strengthen these muscles, which lie deep inside you, it is necessary first of all to locate them. This comes with practice. To find the muscles of the anus, squeeze as if trying to stop a bowel motion. To isolate the muscles of the vagina, pull in and up as though stopping yourself from passing urine. (The front sphincter forms the muscular walls of both the vagina and the urethra and so controls the flow of urine as well as the responsiveness of the vagina.) Locate the anal and vaginal contractions as accurately as possible. When you are tightening the anus alone, relax the vagina. When you are tightening the vaginal/urethra sphincter, relax the anus. When you are contracting both together, be aware of their separate actions. Since the two sphincters form something like a figure-of-eight, it is not in fact possible to completely isolate one or the other and the contraction of either part will have a strengthening effect on the whole. However, aim for as precise a control as you can, paying especial attention to the front sphincter, which is invariably the weaker.

The action in these exercises is one of gripping and lifting, in and up. Whilst you are squeezing, relax completely the surrounding areas – the thighs, abdomen and buttocks. Fine control of the release is as important as the contraction. Let go slowly, very very slowly, and completely. Do not hold any residual tension. Your breathing is especially important during the contractions, because holding the breath can lead to the reverse effect, straining the pelvic floor and encouraging it to droop. (Bearing down as you tighten the muscles has the same effect.) So breathe easily, letting the air come and go. Indeed, holding your breath during *any* exercise can have the effect of straining both the pelvic floor and, if the abdominal muscles are weak, the abdominal wall.

Once you are happy with these pelvic floor contractions they can be done at any time – lying, sitting, walking, talking to friends. Nobody will know you are doing anything at all.

The Benefit
This supremely simple exercise helps to counteract any sagging of the pelvic floor, and so assists proper support of the organs. It can thus be very powerful in helping, or helping to prevent, certain gynaecological and urinary problems, such as prolapse or urinary incontinence. Practised frequently it can also have a near-magical effect on your sex life. The ability to contract consciously during intercourse is an ancient art and, since the pelvic floor forms the muscular walls of the vagina, toning it up will also help the vagina to fit more snugly around the penis, heightening sexual sensation for both partners.

44 The Uplift

Firms bust

Clasp your wrists in front of you at shoulder height. Maintaining the grip and allowing no movement . . . 'push' each hand towards the opposite elbow. Hold. Breathe easily. Press harder. Release. (Repeat with the other hand on top.)

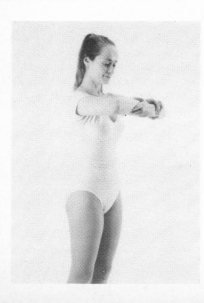

To avoid tension and strain it is important to make sure that your neck is long and straight at the back and that your shoulders are relaxed and low. Hold the left wrist with the right hand and the right with the left, your hands, forearms and elbows lying horizontally at shoulder level. Maintaining the grip, press each hand towards the opposite elbow. No actual movement takes place, but when you are doing it correctly you will feel a strong contraction of the large pectoral muscle.

Hold for about six seconds and then release. Now adjust the height of your hands to the position where you feel that the strongest contraction takes place. That is the position where you will gain maximum benefit. (You may feel a stronger lift by pushing the heels of your hands together. It may feel more effective to push against your upper arms. Find the way which seems best for you, always alternating your hands so each has its turn on top.) Make sure the rest of your body remains quite relaxed throughout. Particularly check any tendency of your head to jerk back or your shoulders to hunch. As in any isometric activity, it is especially important to allow the outbreath. Otherwise you may temporarily raise your blood pressure as well as having aching muscles and feeling very tired.

The Benefit
This is the simplest, the most specific and the best-known bust exercise. It strengthens and improves the tone of the large muscle lying behind the breasts which is chiefly responsible for their shape, position and firmness. So if you despair about being flat-chested this exercise will help make the most of what you have – and perhaps a little more. (On the other hand, it is unlikely actually to make large breasts bigger, as it has no effect on the breast tissue itself, only on muscle.) But whether you are large or small, this exercise can help your shape.

EPILOGUE

In these pages we have proceeded systematically through the body, strengthening some parts and making them firmer and neater, stretching others to release tension and restore flexibility. We have learned to detect and help correct our own particular imbalances, and so to function more freely and effectively. Each of the preceding exercises has its precise purpose and has been designed taking into account the anatomy and mechanics of the human body. No time has been wasted on worse-than-useless workouts.

But, you may still ask, 'Do the exercises *really* work?' My own experience with literally thousands of people provides an unequivocal 'yes'. I could quote example upon example where stiffness has yielded to suppleness or flabbiness to firmness often with a speed which is astonishing.

A case which comes instantly to mind is that of a grandmother whom I shall call Virginia. Virginia had an admirable figure apart from a distinctly bulging abdomen. In three months' time she was to visit family and friends in Australia whom she had not seen for several years, and she was understandably concerned that her unsightly bulge should not travel with her. She made a special arrangement with the health farm where I was working to join, three times a week, the one- and two-week guests in their abdominal exercise classes.

The exercises were those in the abdominal section of this book. Virginia did not go on a diet. Her busy life precluded perfect attendance at the classes and she did not practise at home. She came when she could and worked hard, and long before the three-month deadline she was the envy of the class – the walking proof, the perfect advertisement. She could perform with ease the strongest abdominal exercises which, to their shame, many apparently fit young men could not manage. More to the point was her outline, the sleek new figure that she had so rapidly acquired.

This story illustrates several important features of success. Virginia was highly motivated but not obsessive. Obsession is tension. She worked hard when it was convenient – and in fact she made time to exercise – but she was not compulsive. Many times she abandoned the exercises altogether. Her attitude was relaxed – she enjoyed the classes – and perhaps most telling of all, she visualized herself, quite spontaneously, slim, youthful and elegant.

*

Your body is your way of being in the world. The better it functions, the easier it is for *you* to function. The quality of life is marred by unnecessary physical restriction. The more you are in balance, the freer and stronger your limbs and the straighter your spine, the more will your life be enriched and permeated by a real sense of well-being.

Health and Nutrition from Dent

Holistic Living
A Guide to Self-Care
PATRICK PIETRONI

A revolution is going on in health and healing, in which the emphasis is moving towards an integral approach to ourselves and our surroundings. Dr Patrick Pietroni, Chairman of the British Holistic Medical Association, here introduces the idea of holistic living, and gives guidance on all its important elements – diet and nutrition, stress and how to manage it by exercise, breathing and relaxation, the holistic approach to sex, as well as such key areas as relationships, work and play, the environment and time.

Illustrated throughout with line drawings, the book is full of practical information on self-care and where to find help.

Paperback

Allergic to Food?

A Self-Help Guide

RITA GREER

Food allergy, intolerance or sensitivity has become a fashionable illness and often takes the blame for symptoms caused by entirely different factors – other ilnesses, poor diet or lifestyle. Rita Greer's book puts food allergy into perspective, offering practical help with diagnosis and special diets for the many people for whom self-help may be the only answer.

Paperback

The Good Nutrients Guide

The Complete Handbook of Vitamins, Minerals and Other Nutrients

RITA GREER and ROBERT WOODWARD

This comprehensive handbook, written by a qualified pharmacist and an experienced writer on diet and nutrition, provides an authoritative guide specifically designed for the general consumer. Starting from the idea that nutrients are best when taken in food – although supplements may be useful when this is not practicable – the authors fully describe all the well known vitamins and minerals, as well as the more obscure nutrients, and where necessary give sensible warnings about the overdosing and misdescription of nutrients as 'dietary supplements'. In addition, they give valuable information on relevant legislation and on labelling and other aspects of marketing.

Paperback

The Right Way to Cook

New Recipes for Healthier Living

RITA GREER

The Right Way to Cook is for all those who care about eating healthily *and* want to do so with maximum enjoyment. It provides positive, practical guidance on what we should be eating and how to cook or prepare it – in the most exciting and appetizing way. Starters and snacks, pasta and rice, eggs and vegetarian dishes, fish, meat and poultry, salads, sauces, puddings, bread, cakes, packed meals and celebration food are all covered, and the book also contains menu suggestions and important information on nutrition, shopping and equipment.

Paperback

The Right Way to Eat

To Feel Good – or Even Better

MIRIAM POLUNIN

Does healthy eating mean giving up meat? Does it cost more? Do you need to take vitamin supplements? How much protein do you need? What can better eating do for you – with the minimum of effort? Miriam Polunin's widely acclaimed volume, including a handy up-to-date Appendix of 'E' numbers, is the ideal introduction for everyone in search of clear straightforward advice on eating for better health *and* enhanced well-being.

'The most helpful book on the subject yet to be published. Concise, informative and practical and it spells out the dangers without being alarmist . . . Any parent with young children worried about the dangers of junk food would be well advised to buy this book . . . ' Colin Spencer, *Guardian*

Paperback

Entertaining with Cranks

KAY CANTER and DAPHNE SWANN

An outstanding sequel to the bestselling *The Cranks Recipe Book*

This new volume is full of original recipes especially suitable for celebrating and entertaining. Representing all that is best in gourmet vegetarian cookery, it contains a wide range of delicious and exciting starters and main courses, unusual and imaginative salads, vegetable accompaniments and dressings, and a tempting choice of Cranks famous puddings. The book is lavishly produced and illustrated throughout with John Lawrence's charming pen-and-wash drawings, and 8 pages of colour photographs.

Hardback

The Cranks Recipe Book

DAVID CANTER, KAY CANTER and DAPHNE SWANN

'If you have never bought a book of vegetarian cooking, try this one first.' *Homes and Gardens*

'Inside its homespun linen cover is an unusual cookery book full of good things . . . ' *Daily Telegraph*

'I love their food . . . so I'm delighted that they've brought this book out.' Delia Smith, *Woman's Hour*

'here is a book to delight the eye and the taste buds.' *The Vegetarian*

Hardback

For further information on these titles please contact
The Marketing Department, J. M. Dent & Sons Ltd, Aldine House,
33 Welbeck Street, London W1M 8LX

ORDER FORM

... CANTER & SWANN: Entertaining with Cranks   £12.95
... CANTER, CANTER & SWANN:
    The Cranks Recipe Book   £12.95
... GREER: Allergic to Food?   £2.95
... GREER: The Right Way to Cook   £2.95
... GREER & WOODWARD:
    The Good Nutrients Guide   £3.95
... PIETRONI: Holistic Living   £3.95
... POLUNIN: The Right Way to Eat   £2.50

All these books may be obtained through your local bookshop, or can be ordered direct from the publisher. Please indicate the number of copies required and fill in the form below.

Name .... BLOCK
Address .... LETTERS
.... PLEASE

Please enclose remittance to the value of the cover price *plus* 40p per copy postage to a maximum of £2 for the paperbacks and £1.45 each for the Cranks books, and send your order to:

BP Dept., J. M. Dent & Sons Ltd, 33 Welbeck Street, London W1M 8LX

Applicable to UK only and subject to stock availability